T0184776

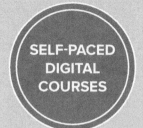
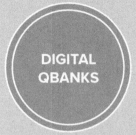
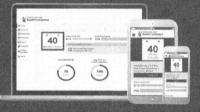
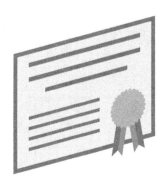
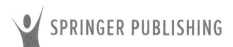

CNOR® CERTIFICATION EXPRESS REVIEW

CNOR® CERTIFICATION EXPRESS REVIEW

SPRINGER PUBLISHING

Springer Publishing Company, LLC
11 West 42nd Street, New York, NY 10036
www.springerpub.com

Acquisitions Editor: Suzanne Toppy
Compositor: diacriTech

ISBN: 978-0-8261-5856-7
ebook ISBN: 978-0-8261-5857-4
DOI: 10.1891/9780826158574

Printed by BnT

The author and the publisher of this Work have made every effort to use sources believed to be reliable to provide information that is accurate and compatible with the standards generally accepted at the time of publication. The author and publisher shall not be liable for any special, consequential, or exemplary damages resulting, in whole or in part, from the readers' use of, or reliance on, the information contained in this book. The publisher has no responsibility for the persistence or accuracy of URLs for external or third-party Internet websites referred to in this publication and does not guarantee that any content on such websites is, or will remain, accurate or appropriate.

Library of Congress Control Number: 2021923767

Contact sales@springerpub.com to receive discount rates on bulk purchases.

Publisher's Note: New and used products purchased from third-party sellers are not guaranteed for quality, authenticity, or access to any included digital components.

Printed in the United States of America.

CONTENTS

PREFACE

If you have purchased this *Express Review*, you are likely well into your exam prep journey to certification. This book was designed to be a high-speed review—a last-minute gut check before your exam day. We created this review, which is a quick summary of the key topics you'll encounter on the exam, to supplement to your certification preparation studies. We encourage you to use it in conjunction with other study aids to ensure you are as prepared as possible for the exam.

This book follows CCI®'s most recent exam content outlines and uses a succinct, bulleted format to highlight what you need to know. The aim of this book is to help you solidify your retention of information in the month or so leading up to your exam. It is written by certified perioperative nurses who are familiar with the exam and the content you need to know. Special features appear throughout the book to call out important information, including:

- **Complications:** Problems that can arise with certain disease states or procedures
- **Pearls:** Additional patient care insights and strategies for knowledge retention
- **Alerts:** Need-to-know details on how to handle emergency situations or when to transfer care
- **Pop Quizzes:** Critical-thinking questions to test your ability to synthesize what you learned (answers in appendix)
- **Unfolding Scenarios:** Case studies that develop over the course of the chapter to challenge your critical-thinking skills (answers in appendix)
- **List of Abbreviations:** A useful appendix to help guide you through the alphabet soup of clinical terms

We know life is busy. Being able to prepare for your exam efficiently and effectively is paramount, which is why we created this *Express Review*. You have come to the right place as you continue on your path of professional growth and development. The stakes are high, and we want to help you succeed. Best of luck to you on your certification journey. You've got this!

PASS GUARANTEE

1

GENERAL EXAMINATION INFORMATION

OVERVIEW

The CNOR® exam is administered by the CCI® to validate basic and advanced knowledge of nurses working in the preoperative, intraoperative, and postoperative phases of surgery. The exam serves as the foundation of established practice and the basis of comparison in future continuing education. Through the successful completion of the exam, the candidate will demonstrate competence in

- The nursing process through the incorporation of critical thinking to engage in safe patient care
- Perioperative nursing practice.

CNOR CERTIFICATION

- The examination is open to all nurses meeting the licensure, continuing education, and experience criteria as set by CCI.
- Once the examination is completed and certification verified, the nurse may utilize CNOR credentialing as a professional designation.
- CCI has been certifying perioperative nurses for over four decades and has certified more than 40,000 perioperative nurses, surgical services managers, perioperative clinical nurse specialists, and other surgery-related nursing specialties worldwide.

ABOUT THE EXAMINATION

- The CNOR examination has 200 multiple choice questions and is 3.75 hr in length.
- Of the 200 multiple choice questions, 185 are scored, and 15 are pretest questions that are not scored.
- The examination blueprint covers the following topics:
  - Pre/Postoperative Patient Assessment and Diagnosis
    - 15% of exam
    - 28 questions
  - Individualized Plan of Care Development and Expected Outcome Identification
    - 8% of exam
    - 15 questions
  - Management of Intraoperative Activities
    - Patient Care and Safety
      - 25% of exam
      - 46 questions
    - Management of Personnel, Services, and Materials
      - 9% of exam
      - 7 questions

(continued)

ABOUT THE EXAMINATION *(continued)*

- Communication and Documentation
  - 11% of exam
  - 20 questions
- Infection Prevention and Control of Environment, Instrumentation, and Supplies
  - 16% of exam
  - 30 questions
- Emergency Situations
  - 10% of exam
  - 18 questions
- Professional Accountabilities
  - 6% of exam
  - 11 questions
- The candidate must correctly answer at least 106 questions to pass the exam.
- Candidates have a 90-day window to take the examination starting the month after application is accepted.
- For information about examination accommodations, review the instructions in the testing handbook.

EXAM ELIGIBILITY

Candidates must meet the following minimum criteria to sit for the exam:
- Hold a license as an RN that is valid in the state or country where they work.
- Be currently working either full or part time in perioperative nursing, nursing education, research, or administration.
- Have at least 2 years of experience in a clinical perioperative setting with at least 1,200 hr working experience as an intraoperative nurse.

HOW TO APPLY

- Candidates may apply by creating an account through CCI at https://www.cc-institute.org/cnor/apply/
  - Include work history, employer contact information, and supervisor contact information.
- Cost of exam: $395.
- Timeline to test:
  - Candidates may schedule the exam Monday through Sunday except for holidays.
  - The 3-month testing window opens the month after candidates' applications have been approved.
  - Once approved, candidates schedule the exam with a PSI testing center in their geographical area.
  - PSI administers the exam. If there is difficulty in locating a PSI testing center, candidates may arrange to take their test via a remote proctor from locations of their choice.

HOW TO RECERTIFY

CNOR certification is active for 5 years. Candidates may recertify by meeting the following requirements:
- Confirm that the following credential and work requirements are met:
  - Hold an active CNOR credential and a current, unrestricted nursing license.
  - Work full or part time in perioperative nursing practice.
  - Attest that a minimum of 500 hr have been worked in perioperative nursing, 250 of which must be in intraoperative care.

- Complete 300 required professional activity points during the 5-year accrual period.
- Submit a renewal application with fee through CCI.
- Candidates who have not completed the required professional activities can apply for a 1-year extension to earn points.

HOW TO CONTACT CCI

- Website: https://www.cc-institute.org/
- Email: info@cc-institute.org
- Certification Administration: (303) 369-9566
- Fax: (303) 695-8464
- Mailing Address:
  Competency and Credentialing Institute
  400 Inverness Pkwy, Suite 265
  Englewood, CO 80112

RESOURCES

Competency & Credentialing Institute. (2021). *CNOR certification & recertification candidate handbook*. https://f.hubspotusercontent30.net/hubfs/2447632/Handbooks/CNOR%20Candidate%20Handbook.pdf
Competency & Credentialing Institute. (n.d.[a]). *CNOR recertification*. https://www.cc-institute.org/cnor/certified-before-2018/
Competency & Credentialing Institute. (n.d.[b]). *CNOR recertification*. https://www.cc-institute.org/cnor/certified-after-2019/

PRE- AND POSTOPERATIVE PATIENT ASSESSMENT AND DIAGNOSIS

OVERVIEW

- A preoperative patient assessment and diagnosis are performed to evaluate issues that pose a significant risk to the patient in the perioperative phase.
- A postoperative patient assessment is performed to evaluate the patient's overall condition and to assess the integrity of the skin and bony prominences immediately following surgical intervention.
- Evaluate for the expected outcomes and use the appropriate interventions if the goal is not achieved.
- *Note:* Throughout each phase of the perioperative experience, the nurse will perform duties using the ACE process:
  - Assess
  - Confirm
  - Evaluate and Ensure

PREOPERATIVE ASSESSMENT

- The preoperative phase of the patient's surgical experience begins upon the decision to have surgery.
- The preoperative assessment is part of the preprocedure verification process, which is the first phase of the Universal Protocol. In this phase of perioperative care, a preprocedure verification is performed to prevent wrong-person, wrong-site, and wrong-procedure occurrences. The preoperative assessment serves the following functions:
  - Identifying patients who are at higher risk for surgical complication associated with the following factors:
    - Age (patients over 65 at greater risk)
    - Alcohol and substance abuse
    - Anticoagulant therapy
    - Diminished activity tolerance
    - High body mass index
    - Invasiveness of the procedure
    - Multiple comorbid conditions
    - Presence of infection
    - Severe or chronic illness
    - Tobacco use
  - Promoting patient safety throughout the perioperative period.
  - Providing the surgical team with the necessary information concerning the patient's baseline health status, which is then used to compare intraoperatively and postoperatively and assess for anomalies.
  - Uncovering comorbidities and other health risks that might contribute to intraoperative complications. Some of the primary comorbidities that contribute to complications are as follows:
    - Cardiovascular disease
    - OSA
    - Reactive airway disease (asthma, COPD)

Assess

- Patient record review
  - Accurate height and weight
  - Allergies and adverse drug reactions
  - Chief complaint
  - History of present illness
- Past medical history
  - Comorbidities such as DM, CAD, COPD, CKD, OSA, clotting disorder, and so on
  - Presence of existing implants
  - Presence of sensory impairment associated with hearing:
    - Adapt communication for the hearing impaired.
    - Explain all actions and interventions being performed.
    - Speak clearly and slowly to ensure that patient can understand and respond appropriately to questions.
  - Presence of visual impairment:
    - Address the patient in a moderate tone and make introductions of the surgical team present.
    - Speak to the patient before touching to avoid startling them.
  - Presence of impairment associated with cognitive function:
    - Explain interventions at the patient's level of understanding.
    - Use simple phrases to convey instruction.
  - Preexisting medical conditions that can increase the risk of fluid and electrolyte imbalance:
    - Burn-related injuries
    - Liver disease
    - Renal disease
- Past surgical history (e.g., prior surgeries, mastectomy, implanted stimulators, MH)
- Medication review
  - Medication reconciliation present on the chart
  - Report of last medications taken and time taken (beta-blockers within the last 24 hr, administration of prophylactic antibiotics, antimicrobial bathing, etc.)
  - That all aspects of the medication reconciliation are complete, to include the following:
    - Name, dose, frequency, route, and purpose of all drugs taken regularly
    - Standardized method for reporting the information to other members of the healthcare team
- Family history
  - Report of significant family history (history of heart disease, clotting disorder, etc.)
- Social history
  - Alcohol use or history of alcohol use
  - Diet and diet restrictions associated with preexisting conditions
  - Illicit drug use or history of illicit drug use
  - Exercise routine
- Cultural assessment
  - Evaluation of the patient's cultural background, education, and cultural needs
  - Examination and accommodation of patient's religious beliefs
  - Use of translation services if needed
- Functional assessment
  - Age-specific psychosocial assessment
  - Basic evaluation of the patient's physical strength and pulses
  - Complications with range of motion that may limit procedural positioning needs
  - Patient's ability to perform activities of daily living
  - Sensory deficits and neurologic function
- Review of systems
  - Review of systems conducted by the preadmission testing office and anesthesia personnel

- Physical exam
  - Patient's pain level
    - ○ Communicate patient's report of pain level to the anesthesia personnel, surgeon, and surgical team.
    - ○ Consider the neurologic function and level of consciousness during the pain assessment.
    - ○ Use a standardized method for charting the patient's pain level.
  - Patient's skin
    - ○ Assess the integrity of skin, looking for bruising, skin tears, signs of infection, and scarring.
- Laboratory and diagnostic tests may include some of the following and will be ordered by either the surgeon, anesthesiologist, or both depending on the patient's surgery and comorbidities:
  - Labs
    - ○ BMP
    - ○ CBC
    - ○ Creatinine
    - ○ INR
    - ○ LFT
    - ○ PT
    - ○ PTT
    - ○ Type and screen
  - Radiology
    - ○ CT Scan
    - ○ MRI results
    - ○ Ultrasound
    - ○ X-ray
  - Other diagnostics
    - ○ EKG
    - ○ Pregnancy test
    - ○ Urinalysis

NURSING PEARL

SAMPLE Mnemonic

Rothrock identified the mnemonic, SAMPLE, as a quick guide used to gather the pertinent history. In emergent situations, this may be gathered after the surgical intervention has begun.

- **S**ymptoms
- **A**llergies
- **M**edications
- **P**ast medical history
- **L**ast oral intake
- **E**vents or **E**nvironment that led to the accident or injury

UNFOLDING SCENARIO 2.1A

A 54-year-old female patient is scheduled for hysteroscopy with dilation and curettage. Patient education was provided related to lithotomy positioning and expectations after the procedure. Piercings have been removed. The patient denies alcohol or drug use and is a nonsmoker. The patient has been NPO since midnight and took only lisinopril 10 mg with a sip of water this morning. The patient reports having lumbar fusion and low back pain. The patient weighs 152 lb. and is 5 ft. 4 in. tall. Warm blankets have been placed on the patient.

Question

What other aspects of the preoperative assessment are necessary?

Confirm

- Informed consent
  - The patient has been informed as to the following:
    - ○ Description of the procedure and alternative therapies
    - ○ Explanation of risks associated with the procedure
    - ○ Explanation that the patient has the right to refuse treatment or withdraw consent
    - ○ Name and qualifications of the person(s) performing the procedure
    - ○ Underlying disease process and natural course
  - The patient has no questions related to the planned procedure.
  - The patient (or their representative) has signed (on paper or electronically) verifying consent to the surgical procedure.

(continued)

Confirm *(continued)*

- Patient identification
  - If the patient is suffering from cognitive impairment or cannot verbalize name and date of birth, the patient's identity verification process should be performed per the organization's policy and procedure.
  - In some cases, the patient medical record number will also be checked if the organization is utilizing barcode medication scanning.
- Code status per AORN
  - Confirm that the advanced directive or do-not-resuscitate order (where applicable) is complete and present on the patient's chart:
    - *Allow Natural Death Orders:* A directive written by a physician to promote a discussion related to end-of-life care decisions
    - *Do Not Intubate or Do Not Resuscitate:* A special directive stating that no cardiopulmonary resuscitation be performed
    - *Full Code:* The performance of full cardiopulmonary resuscitation efforts
- Correct procedure and site marking
  - Confirm the site is marked with a marker that will withstand the prep solution of choice so that the mark is apparent and visible to all team members after preparation. Ensure that all consents are in the chart and that they are signed.
- Surgical environment
  - Confirm the OR is stocked with the following basic room contents:
    - Anesthesia machine and supplies
    - Biohazard receptacle
    - ESU
    - Instrument table
    - Kick bucket
    - Linen hamper
    - Mayo stand
    - Other supplies and equipment as required by the procedure
    - OR bed or table
    - Prep table
    - Sharps container
    - Suction apparatus and supplies
    - Trash bin
  - Cleanliness of suite
    - Preliminary cleaning with FDA-approved disinfectant. Ensure that at the start of the day, preliminary cleaning with an FDA-approved cleaning agent (known as damp dusting) was performed.
- Specimen management needs
  - Collaboration with the surgeon to address the prospective specimen to be collected, handling, and disposition
  - Need for photography equipment (e.g., Mohs procedures)
  - Specimen collection equipment

 ALERT!

The perioperative nurse may serve as the witness to consent. It is the nurse's function to ensure that the patient can verbalize understanding of the procedure to be performed and has no questions. All documents (such as the surgical consent, advance directive, and do-not-resuscitate order) must be fully executed before the patient can be taken to the surgical suite for the procedure.

Evaluate and Ensure

- Ensure there are no barriers to completing a perioperative assessment, such as the following:
  - Emergent situations.
  - NPO status (or lack thereof) can cause surgery cancellation or delay.

- Language barriers can cause a delay in the procedure due to a need to access an interpreter.
- Cultural barriers can create communication barriers and delay the procedure.
- Cognitive impairment can create communication barriers.
- Missing test results, history, and physical assessment can create delays in the scheduled procedure time.
- Ensure that the patient has received adequate education:
  - Answer any last-minute questions and ensure the patient and family member(s) verbalize understanding of the procedure.
  - Patient education must be tailored to the patient's age, readiness to learn, level of learning, and culture.
  - Teaching materials should be provided to patients and their family members and written at the patient's level of literacy.
- Ensure family/contact presence:
  - Make sure there is an up-to-date contact number in the chart so that the surgeon may update the appropriate family member/friend intra- and postop.
- Ensure the following last-minute considerations:
  - A urinary catheter has been placed, if indicated.
  - Active type and screen, appropriate blood products have been typed and crossed and are available in the blood bank.
  - All personal articles have been removed.
  - Any diagnostic tests/lab results are available in the chart.
  - Normothermia measures (blankets, forced-air warmers) are in place for perioperative and postoperative implementation.
  - Special equipment available.
  - The patient has been NPO since midnight.

POP QUIZ 2.1

A 56-year-old male is admitted through the preoperative patient holding area for left shoulder arthroplasty. The nurse is performing the preoperative assessment and notices that the surgical site has not been marked. The anesthesiologist is set up to perform a scalene nerve block. What should the nurse do?

UNFOLDING SCENARIO 2.1B

After the patient has been intubated and anesthesia has commenced, the patient is positioned on the OR table and legs placed in the padded stirrups. The safety belt is securely strapped across the patient's abdomen at the request of the surgeon. The sterile draping and surgical prep are applied by the scrub technician.

Question

What is the circulating nurse's next course of action?

INTRAOPERATIVE ASSESSMENT AND UNIVERSAL PROTOCOL

- The intraoperative phase begins when the patient is transferred onto the OR bed or table.
- The perioperative nurse uses the nursing process to guide nursing practice and enhance perioperative assessment.
- The Universal Protocol starts in the preoperative phase; however, it is centered around the time-out process, which occurs in the intraoperative phase.
- The Universal Protocol is a safety practice developed by TJC that begins in the preoperative phase and continues during the intraoperative phase. It consists of the following:
  - Conducting a preprocedure verification process
  - Marking the surgical site as appropriate
  - Performing the time-out

Assess

- Preprocedure verification process:
  - Verify the correct procedure, patient, and site (involve the patient when necessary).
  - Identify the items needed for the procedure (implants, equipment, instrumentation, medications, personnel).
  - Utilize a standardized list to verify the availability of items needed for the procedure.
- Patient setup:
  - Place the patient on the OR table.
  - Assist anesthesia personnel with proper connection of monitoring; the anesthesia personnel may intubate the patient, place a central line, and place an arterial line.
  - Set up medication, to include priming of appropriate medications and IV pump setup, having emergency medications prepared, and so on.
  - Maintain patient privacy.
  - Clear pathway around the sterile field.
  - Insert urinary catheter (if not already done during preop).
  - Position patient for specific procedure and ensure patient is properly secured with appropriate safety straps.
  - Clip hair at the surgical site if ordered.
  - Prepare the surgical site with chlorhexidine or other solution as ordered.
- Type of wound closure to be performed:
  - *Primary intention:* Characterized by wounds created under sterile conditions, minimal tissue destruction present with edges of wounds approximated
  - *Secondary intention:* Characterized by chronic, dirty, or infected wounds not closed and allowed to heal through granulation
  - *Delayed primary closure or tertiary intention:* Characterized by wounds requiring debridement and delayed healing of 3 days or more after injury or surgical intervention
- Wound management
  - *Debridement:* Removal of devitalized tissue from the wound through sharp excision, mechanical irrigation, enzymatic agents, or biological methods
  - Hydrotherapy or hydrosurgery
    - Hydrotherapy is frequently used in the OR and is referred to as pulsatile lavage.
    - Hydrosurgery is performed using pressurized irrigation and localized vacuum to remove devitalized tissue.
  - *Hyperbaric oxygenation:* Use of a hyperbaric chamber to increase oxygenation to the wound. The chamber can also encourage cellular regeneration for chronic wounds.
  - *Negative-pressure wound therapy:* Use of a vacuum-assisted closure device, drainage sponge, and occlusive dressing for the long-term management of chronic or nonhealing wounds.
- Risk factors
  - Blood loss likely during surgical event.
  - Arthroscopic surgery requires introduction of an increased amount of normal saline to the surgical site for visualization (fluid can leech into the surrounding tissues and vasculature).

 ALERT!

TJC identified that in the case of an unconscious patient, the nurse should follow the policy established by the facility related to the identification process. Further, TJC also identified that the facility may use temporary names until family members identify the patient.

 NURSING PEARL

AORN Wound Classification
- *Class I:* Class I includes clean wounds that are not infected and show no signs of inflammation.
- *Class II:* Clean-contaminated wounds are associated with the respiratory, alimentary, or genitourinary tract where no infection or break in aseptic technique is present.
- *Class III:* Contaminated wounds are related to accidents, penetrating trauma, fractures, and operations with multiple breaks in aseptic technique. Some signs of infection and gross spillage of infectious material may be present.
- *Class IV:* Dirty or infected wounds are traumatic and contain retained devitalized tissue. The wound contains infectious material.

- Abdominal surgery involving the bowel or pancreas can cause third spacing.
- Gastrointestinal surgery can cause bowel preparation (associated presentation of dehydration).
- Neurosurgery causes dysregulation of antidiuretic hormone and hyponatremia.
- Vaginal hysteroscopy requires introduction of sterile fluids to improve visualization of the pelvic organs (fluids can leech into the surrounding tissues and vasculature).
- Fluid overload or excessive loss can occur through the following:
  - Cell damage related to manipulation during surgery
  - Drains
  - Nasogastric tube suctioning
  - Prolonged surgery time
  - Stoma leakage
- Assess the placement of dispersive electrode grounding pad (Bovie pad).
  - Protect the patient from electric shock or burns by placing a dispersive electrode grounding pad on the patient.
  - Avoid placement of the grounding pad on hair, bony prominences, dry skin, or adipose tissue.
  - Place the adhesive side of the grounding pad on an area of the body that is
    - as far away from an implanted pacemaker or ICD as possible,
    - flush to the skin and not tented,
    - not over any metal implants or prosthesis (e.g., hip implants, knee implants, rods),
    - on an area that has muscle mass and vascularity, and
    - opposite of the surgical site.
  - Plug the pad into the ESU, and position the ESU on the same side as the primary surgeon where the settings can be visualized.
  - Confirm current type to be used with the surgeon.

Special Considerations

1. Pediatric patient assessment considerations:
   - Airway and lungs
     - Infants are obligate nose breathers, and the respiratory muscle fatigues easily.
     - The airway is considerably smaller, and there is increased airway resistance.
     - The epiglottis is floppy, and the glottis is more anterior, making intubation more challenging.
   - Cardiovascular
     - Evaluation of any cardiovascular anomalies is vital due to the effects that anesthetic agents have on vasodilation and the contractility of the heart.
     - Infants have decreased cardiac compliance.
     - Young children are predisposed to increased vagal tone that is often induced by painful stimuli.
   - Fluid management
     - Infants and young children have immature kidney function and are prone to dehydration.
   - Metabolism
     - Infants have a high basal rate.
     - Children younger than 2 years have immature liver function and protein binding.
     - Delivery of medication should be titrated based on age, weight, and overall health.
   - Temperature regulation
     - Exposure to extremes of cold and hot should be prevented.
     - Infants and younger children are at high risk for hypothermia due to the low body surface area ratio and thin adipose tissue layer.
     - Only the surgical area should be exposed to prevent hypothermia.

 ALERT!

TJC Universal Protocol Standard UP0101: Element of Performance 1 requires that a preprocedure process is performed to verify the correct procedure, patient, and site. The patient should be involved in this process whenever possible.

(continued)

Special Considerations (continued)

- Skin and prep solutions
  - ○ Use caution with CHG- and alcohol-based preoperative patient skin prep due to the potential for chemical burns.
  - ○ Use caution with povidone-iodine-based solutions due to the risk of iodine poisoning.
2. Trauma surgery and ATLS assessment considerations:
   - Upon transfer of the patient from the emergency department to the perioperative suite, the following should occur:
     - ○ Assess the patient's airway, respiratory function, and circulation.
     - ○ Assess the level of neurologic disability.
     - ○ Examine the extent of the injuries and thermoregulation of the patient.
   - After the preliminary assessment is complete, a secondary assessment is performed:
     - ○ Assist anesthesia personnel with acquiring vital signs, connection to monitoring, procurement of laboratory specimens, and other life-supporting interventions.
     - ○ Assist surgeon with a physical inspection of the entirety of the patient's body.
     - ○ Ensure family/contact presence.
     - ○ Connect the family with the OR navigator (if one is used) or the waiting area staff.
     - ○ Provide the family with an overview of the status of the patient and advise that the surgeon will explain the surgical procedure to be performed.
     - ○ Management of uncontrolled bleeding will require the following interventions by the surgical team, such as the following:
       - ■ Application of pressure directly to the bleeding site
       - ■ Application of pressure over arterial sites
     - ○ Assist in the administration of blood and blood products.
     - ○ Collaborate with the surgeon and anesthesia team related to interventions associated with cardiovascular and blood volume changes.
     - ○ Elevate extremities as appropriate.
     - ○ Expedite laboratory processing of samples.
     - ○ Monitor intake and output during the surgical procedure.
     - ○ The acquisition of the history and physical may be provided by the patient, but in extreme cases may need to be acquired from the family member. In emergent conditions where the patients cannot identify themselves, such as in trauma, the patient will be identified according to the process outlined in the facility policy.

Confirm

- Conduct the time-out immediately before the invasive procedure or before the incision is made. All team members must agree on the correct patient identity, site, procedure to be done, administration of antibiotics (if required), and confirmation that all items needed for surgery are present in the surgical suite.
- Verify correct site marking, as noted preoperatively.
- Confirm patient safety measures have been performed (e.g., placement of the safety strap).
- Confirm combined roles/duties of the scrub and circulating nurse have been performed:
  - Ensure that any contamination encountered during the procedure has been confined and contained.
  - Perform a surgical count at the beginning and the end of the procedure, as well as any time a count is called for during the procedure.
  - Ensure that all surgical team members are aware that a surgical count has taken place and the result of said count is communicated.
  - All activity must cease in the event that there is an incorrect count.

 ALERT!

AORN recommends that the perioperative nurse functions as a patient advocate and communicates with all members of the surgical team and other nursing personnel to ensure that all the components of the universal protocol have been addressed.

- Work collaboratively with the surgeon and anesthesia team to promote positive patient outcomes.
- Confirm specific roles/duties of the scrub nurse have been performed:
  - Collaborates with circulating nurse to set up OR suite for procedure
  - Collaborates with surgeon related to procedural needs
  - Drapes all tables, stands, and sterile field
  - Ensures ESU pencil or other apparatus safely stowed when not in use and ensures tip is kept clean
  - Ensures that sterility of surgical field is maintained, instrumentation passed in safe manner, all sharps and sponges accounted for, and patient safety preserved
  - Establishes baseline counts for all sponges, sharps, and other countable materials used
  - Gowns members of surgical team
  - Labels medications
  - Maintains sterile technique during procedure
  - Manages sterile field and breaches in technique
  - Passes all cords off in one direction if possible
  - Prepares hemostatic agents as required for procedure
  - Prepares sterile instruments and supplies
  - Prevents retained foreign objects in patient
  - Positions all tables, stands, and equipment after draping
  - Reconciles count
  - Safely handles and manages all sharps, sutures, and other related closure materials
  - Sets up drains and dressings
  - Validates medications dispensed to sterile field
- Confirm specific roles/duties of the circulating nurse have been completed:
  - Applies dispersive electrode pad
  - Assists with OR suite preparation
  - Assists with transfer of patient
  - Assists anesthesia personnel during induction and intraoperatively (as needed)
  - Checks all case items/equipment and compares against physician preference list
  - Charges patient for only items used
  - Collaborates with all surgical team members to promote patient outcomes and safety
  - Coordinates connection of equipment adjacent to sterile field
  - Documents all patient care and interventions according to facility policy and procedure
  - Ensures the pathway around sterile field perimeter is clear and safety hazards have been addressed (cords, equipment, foot pedals, etc.)
  - Initiates time-out
  - Inspects all package integrity
  - Maintains accountability for instruments, sponges, sharps, and specimen handling
  - Monitors for breaches in technique
  - Obtains and dispenses solutions to sterile field using continuous motion to avoid aerosolization
  - Opens all sterile supplies with assistance from surgical scrub person or other facilitating nurse
  - Performs ongoing evaluation of patient's fluid output and notes/advises surgical team of the following:
    - Blood loss: Surgical sponges removed from the field and fluid capture through suction canisters should be monitored throughout the procedure.

 ALERT!

There are three types of hazards in OR environment:
- *Biological:* Pathogenic organisms, infectious waste, needlesticks or cuts, and latex sensitivity
- *Chemical:* Anesthesia gas exposure, toxic fumes or electrocautery plume, cytotoxic drugs, and cleaning agents
- *Physical:* Falls, noise, irradiation, and fire

(continued)

Confirm *(continued)*

- ○ Fluid amounts: The bags of fluid used during the procedure must be accounted for and the surgical team made aware of the number of bags. For hysteroscopy, endoscopic, or urologic procedures, ensure the patient is in the appropriate position and the amount of fluid administered is closely monitored to prevent fluid overload.
- Performs skin asepsis as directed by surgeon or ensures that skin asepsis performed correctly
- Positions OR bed corresponding to overhead lighting
- Prepares medications for dispensation to field
- Pretests equipment
- Promotes a culture of safety and advocates for patient
- Performs handoff reporting to recovery room nurse
- Tests overhead lights, suction, and other equipment as appropriate
- Validates implants

 UNFOLDING SCENARIO 2.1C

After the patient has been intubated and anesthesia commenced, the patient is positioned on the OR table with their torso, neck, and head in the supine position and legs placed in the padded stirrups. The sterile draping is about to be applied when the circulating nurse notices that the safety strap is laying on the floor. The anesthesia personnel confirm that the arm straps are secure on both arms.

Question

What is the circulating nurse's next course of action?

Evaluate and Ensure

- Instrument sterility using Spaulding classification system:
  - Critical: Must be sterile and will enter tissue or vascular system (instruments, cutting endoscopic accessories, needles)
  - Semi-critical: Should be sterile but high-level disinfection acceptable according to manufacturer's IFU (anesthesia equipment, endoscopes)
  - Noncritical: Intermediate- to low-level disinfection or cleaning required (OR beds and linens, patient care items)
  - Sterility maintained using aseptic technique when dispensing materials and instruments to sterile field
- Surgical environment safety check preventing slips and falls:
  - Arrange equipment and supplies to promote an unobstructed path.
  - Limit traffic and provide clear pathways in the suite.
  - Post signage where wet floors are present.
  - Rapidly clean up spills and debris.
  - Reduce clutter and cords on the floor.
  - Wear slip-resistant footwear and shoe covers.
- Intraoperative complication evaluation:
  - Deep vein thrombosis symptoms (most commonly seen postoperatively)
  - Respiratory complications:
    - ○ Carbon dioxide accumulation
    - ○ Ineffective oxygenation
    - ○ Intraabdominal pressure from positioning or insufflation

 ALERT!

TJC Universal Protocol Standard UP0101: Element of Performance 2 requires that relevant documentation and all labeled diagnostic and radiology test results are appropriately displayed in the surgical suite. Additionally, this element of performance requires that blood products, implantable materials and devices, and other special equipment are available for the procedure.

- Pain sensation, which can be noted by hypertension and tachycardia
- Bruising
- Red or darkened skin
- Swollen veins
- Warmth and tenderness at the site
- Hematoma
  - Abnormal collection of blood within a tissue space
- Hypovolemia
  - Possible causes of hypovolemia:
    - Gastric or nasogastric tube aspirate
    - Intraoperative fluid and blood loss (i.e., hemorrhage)
    - Wound drainage
  - Signs and symptoms of hypovolemia:
    - Decreased urine output
    - Sunken fontanels (infants)
    - Tachycardia
    - Uncontrolled bleeding
- Hypervolemia
  - Possible causes of hypervolemia:
    - Decreased urine output
    - Impaired kidney and cardiac function
    - Retained irrigation
  - Signs and symptoms of hypervolemia:
  - Engorged varicose veins
    - Hypertension
    - Neck vein distention
    - Pitting edema
    - Tachycardia
    - Tachypnea
- Vital sign changes dependent on clinical status, specific surgery performed, and presence of comorbidities may occur intraoperatively but is medically managed by anesthesia team collaboration with surgeon:
  - Arrhythmias
  - Bradycardia
  - Fever
  - Hypertension
  - Hypotension
  - Oxygen saturation
  - Tachycardia

POP QUIZ 2.2

A 67-year-old female is admitted through the preoperative patient holding area for a right knee arthroscopy. A right femoral nerve block was administered by anesthesia personnel in the preoperative holding area to save time. While moving the patient from the stretcher to the surgical table, the nurse notices that the surgeon marked the left knee. What is the most appropriate action for the circulating nurse?

POSTOPERATIVE ASSESSMENT

- The postoperative assessment is performed, in varying degrees, by the entire surgical team.
- Postoperatively, the patient is admitted either to the postanesthesia care unit or the intensive care unit, depending upon the patient's acuity.

Assess

- Perform a postop assessment:
  - Assess vital signs frequently depending on type of anesthesia need (e.g., local only), clinical status, and institutional guidelines.
    - Warming device if patient is hypothermic

(continued)

Assess *(continued)*

- ○ When nurse is serving as the local anesthesia nurse
  - ■ assess for hemodynamic stability, respiratory status, and need for supplemental oxygen;
  - ■ continuously monitor EKG if necessary.
- Evaluate the patient's pain level. Administer pharmacologic agents as ordered.
- Assess for skin integrity.
  - ○ Appearance of bruising, skin tears, signs of infection, and scarring
  - ○ Bony prominences for pressure injuries
  - ○ Skin cleanliness
  - ○ Clean, dry, intact dressings
- If the wound is uncovered, assess the wound closure (closed and intact, or open for healing by secondary intention).
- Evaluate for wound healing complications.
  - ○ Separation: Wound edges begin to come apart
  - ○ Dehiscence: Separation of fascial layer with development of drainage
  - ○ Evisceration: Surgical emergency where abdominal contents spill out of abdominal cavity
- Consider during the recovery period:
  - Can the patient have food and drink if recovering well postop?
  - Is the patient waking up appropriately from anesthesia?
  - If the patient is intubated, are they reversed (if paralyzed)?
  - Does the surgeon want postop labs sent?
  - Does the patient need blood products?
- Some facilities may require frequent assessments including the use of the Aldrete scoring system (measurement of recovery after anesthesia). Use the appropriate postop protocol for the institution.

Confirm

- Actions to occur at the end of the procedure:
  - Provide assistance to anesthesia personnel during the extubation of the patient, if indicated.
  - Ensure that dressings are applied by appropriate scrubbed staff (nurse, technician, RNFA, PA, NP, surgeon).
  - Ensure the patient is safely repositioned to a supine position with assistance.
  - Ensure the transfer of the patient to the stretcher or bed is performed by at least four people.
- Specimen procurement and confirmation:
  - Specimen procurement and confirmation will be completed by the circulating nurse and scrub personnel through the following actions:
    - ○ Assist the surgeon in receiving verbal confirmation of the diagnosis or specimen-related details with the pathologist (related to specimens sent for frozen section).
    - ○ Label accurately.
    - ○ Minimize the risk of specimen compromise through careful transfer from the sterile field.
    - ○ Reduce the number of people involved in the specimen handling process.
    - ○ Use a dedicated space for specimen management on and off the sterile field.
    - ○ Verify the patient identification and specimen identification on the label with the read-back method to review specimen names and disposition has been performed.
    - ○ Confirm the procedure performed is recorded in the patient's health record.
    - ○ Deviations from the primary scheduled procedure can occur and are related to complications experienced during surgery.
- Surgical counts
  - Ensure that surgical counts (sponges, instruments, sharps, and any other materials) have been completed and the surgical team has been made aware of any discrepancies. If there is a discrepancy noted, follow the institutional policy for discrepancy resolution and documentation.
  - Ensure the following actions are done related to the care of the patient:

- ○ Normothermia is maintained by placing warm blankets (or forced-air warming) on the patient immediately following the application of dressings.
  - ○ Maintain the position of drains (if used). Ensure drains that have not moved are appropriately secured, if applicable.
- Cleaning with FDA-approved disinfectant at the end of the procedure:
  - Place biohazardous material in the appropriate receptacle following the procedure.
  - Dispose sharps in the appropriate containers.
  - Dispose solutions and suction container contents according to the facility policy.

Evaluate and Ensure

- Ensure the following actions have occurred at the end of the procedure:
  - All contaminated items are removed.
  - Drains are appropriately secured, draining, and patent.
  - Patient is positioned back on bed safely.
  - Family has been updated.
  - Nonradiopaque sponges are removed.
  - Normothermia is maintained.
- Evaluation of the patient's clinical status:
  - Extubation readiness (per surgeon and anesthesia personnel)
  - Recovery need evaluation of patient (PACU or ICU) based on patient's clinical status and recommendations of surgery and anesthesia team
- Effective communication and handoff reporting to receiving unit:
  - Postop report process specific to facility
    - ○ Often performed with all members of surgical team:
      - Anesthesia personnel: Patient's vital signs, medications administered, blood loss, complications, and pain level
      - Circulating nurse: Surgical procedure performed, identification of drains or tubes, type of dressing used, and presence of other supportive medical equipment (braces, slings, blood salvage, and safety concerns)
      - Surgeon: What was done during the procedure
    - ○ Alternatively performed with anesthesia and/or surgery personnel:
      - Circulating nurse may stay in surgical suite to promote faster turnover and call receiving RN, reporting patient's condition, position of drains, type of dressing, need for additional equipment, and other patient care needs.

NURSING PEARL

Wound Healing Phases
- *Inflammatory:* This phase lasts 0 to 3 days with redness, edema, and phagocytosis occurring.
- *Proliferation:* This phase lasts 4 to 24 days with granulation and epithelial tissue forming.
- *Maturation:* This phase lasts 24 days to 1 year with scar formation and contracture of tissue forming.

POP QUIZ 2.3

A 77-year-old male is admitted through the preoperative patient holding area for a right total knee arthroplasty. The patient sustained blood loss associated with injury to the popliteal artery. The patient will likely need a blood transfusion postoperatively. To promote continuity of care, what should the circulating nurse report to the PACU nurse?

UNFOLDING SCENARIO 2.1D

After the procedure, the circulating nurse notices that hysteroscopy irrigation has leaked on the floor and is not part of the output volume collected in the suction canister. While repositioning the patient from lithotomy to supine position with assistance from the scrub technician, the circulating nurse notices that the patient's legs are edematous. The surgeon has already left the room.

Question
What is the circulating nurse's next course of action?

UNFOLDING SCENARIO 2.2A

A 58-year-old female patient is scheduled for a laparoscopic low anterior bowel resection related to a cancerous tumor found on a CT scan. The following are the preoperative assessment findings.

- Paperwork
  - All paperwork (anesthesia consent, surgical consent, history and physical, and associated laboratory and diagnostic workup) are present.
- Vital signs
  - *Initial vital signs are EKG:* NSR, BP 110/60, HR 72, 16; SpO_2 100%.
  - The patient is intubated with a 7.0-mm endotracheal tube without difficulty. Preoperatively, a 20-gauge IV is placed in the right antecubital fossa. The cystic artery is cut, and the laparoscopic bowel resection is emergently converted to an open procedure. An additional 16-gauge IV has been placed in the left antecubital fossa; both IVs are wide open with fluids being administered. An esophageal temperature probe has been inserted. An arterial line has been inserted into the right radial artery. Current fluid volume deficit indicators are thready pulse, decreased venous filling, and decreased cardiac output.
- Lab values show two critical issues. Here are the Baseline Laboratory Results:
  - *WBC 9.7 103/µL Reference range:* 4.0 to 11.0
  - *RBC 5.5 106/µL Reference range:* 4.6 to 6.2
  - *HGB 11.0 g/dL Reference range:* 12.0 to 15.0
  - *HCT 34 % Reference range:* 36 to 46
  - *PLT 410 cells/µL Reference range:* 140 to 450
  - No pregnancy test performed due to patient hysterectomy at age 50 years
- History and physical
  - Patient education was provided related to the possibility of repositioning during the procedure to lithotomy to improve access and associated with the surgeon's surgical approach.
  - Piercings have been removed.
  - The patient denies alcohol or drug use and is a nonsmoker.
  - The patient is married and has two children.
  - The patient is a Jehovah's Witness and has declined to sign the blood consent.
  - The patient has been NPO since midnight and took only metoprolol 25 mg with a sip of water in the morning.
  - The patient reported a scar associated with a cesarean section 20 years ago.
  - The patient weighs 145 lb. and is 5 ft. 4 in. tall.

Question

What other aspects of the assessment are necessary?

UNFOLDING SCENARIO 2.2B

The surgeon begins to perform the bowel resection and notices that there are multiple adhesions wrapped around the area of the bowel to be resected. The surgeon begins to perform soft dissection to gently remove the adhesions when the bowel perforates. Gross fecal spillage from the intestine begins to fill the abdominal cavity, and the patient begins to hemorrhage.

Question

What is the circulating nurse's next course of action both off and on the sterile field?

UNFOLDING SCENARIO 2.2C

The anesthesiologist alerts the surgeon that the patient has become tachycardic and asks how much blood was lost. The circulating nurse verbalizes to the team the volume of blood and fluid collected in the suction canister (3L). The circulator reminds the team that the patient is a Jehovah's Witness and refused to sign the blood consent, even though patient education from the surgeon and anesthesiologist was provided.

The surgeon successfully stops the bleeding and resects the bowel. The surgical cavity is irrigated. The anesthesiologist pages the chief of anesthesia to take over for the anesthesiologist of record, who left to consult the patient's family. The anesthesiologist of record returns to the room stating that he received consent for blood products and transfusion from the patient's husband, who is listed as the medical decision-maker in the living will on the chart.

Question

What is the circulating nurse's next course of action related to the transfusion?

RESOURCES

Association for periOperative Registered Nurses. (2015). *Position statement: Preventing wrong-patient, wrong-site, wrong-procedure events.* https://www.aorn.org/guidelines/clinical-resources/tool-kits/correct-site-surgery-tool-kit

Association for periOperative Registered Nurses. (2016). *AORN Perioperative efficiency toolkit.* https://www.aorn. org/-/media/aorn/guidelines/tool-kits/perioperative-efficiency/aorn-perioperative-efficiency-tool-kit-webinar. pdf?la=en

Association for periOperative Registered Nurses. (2019). *Guideline essentials: Key takeaways. Team Communication.* https://www.aorn.org/essentials/team-communication

Caple, C. R. B. M., & Kornusky, J. R. M. (2018). *Preoperative assessment: Performing.* CINAHL nursing guide. EBSCO.

The Joint Commission. (2021b). *What are the key elements organizations need to understand regarding the use of two patient identifiers prior to providing care, treatment or services?* https://www.jointcommission.org/standards/standard-faqs/home-care/national-patient-safety-goals-npsg/000001545/

The Joint Commission. (2021a). *The universal protocol.* https://www.jointcommission.org/standards/universal-protocol/Phillips, N., & Hornacky, A. (2021). *Berry and Kohn's operating room technique* (14th ed.). Elsevier.

Rothrock, J. C., & McEwen, D. R. (2019). *Alexander's care of the patient in surgery* (16th ed.). Elsevier.

3

INDIVIDUALIZED PLANS OF CARE AND EXPECTED OUTCOMES

OVERVIEW

- A perioperative nurse should develop comprehensive plans of care spanning the preoperative, intraoperative, and postoperative phases of the surgical experience using an evidence-based practice approach that follows the nursing process and incorporates PNDS standard nursing language.
- Each patient's plan of care is individualized based on patient-specific assessment data. This ensures the best patient outcomes and highest quality care.
- The perioperative nurse uses NANDA guidance to formulate nursing diagnoses associated with the individualized plan of care.
- Evidence-based practice approaches in developing plans of care include the use of the AORN Guidelines for Perioperative Practice.
- Each guideline summarizes research and nonresearch evidence supporting best practices around a clinical question or topic guiding the selection of nursing interventions that lead to expected patient outcomes.

MEASURABLE PATIENT OUTCOMES

- In this section, standards of perioperative nursing, the use of standardized nursing language, surgical conscience, and fostering a culture of safety are discussed as each relates to the perioperative nurses' role in achieving measurable patient outcomes.
- The achievement of positive patient outcomes is central to nursing practice.

Standards of Perioperative Nursing

- According to AORN Guidelines for Perioperative Practice, the perioperative nurse should perform the following:
  - Acquire specialized knowledge associated with the various types of surgical services.
  - Adhere to ethical principles and standards of practice.
  - Advocate for patients.
  - Collaborate with all members of the surgical team to promote positive patient outcomes.
  - Collect data and documents thoroughly in the legal health record.
  - Contribute to personal growth and the development of the self and peers.
  - Cultivate a healthy work environment.
  - Identify trends related to quality, patient safety, and provision of care.
  - Incorporate research into practice.
  - Provide leadership in the practice setting.
  - Systematically review the quality of care.
  - Use standardized nursing language in the documentation and planning of patient care.
  - Utilize resources in a cost-efficient manner.
- The standards of perioperative nursing are focused on the provision of nursing care and the roles of the nurse. The standards apply to all nurses.
- The standards are developed by AORN and align with the American Nurses Association's scope and standards of practice.

Standardized Nursing Language

- The AORN developed the PNDS, a standardized nomenclature, to support perioperative nursing practice across the continuum. The nurse selects PNDS data elements and definitions as appropriate to influence patient outcomes.
- An example of an outcome statement using the PNDS is: The patient will be free from signs and symptoms of surgical infection.

Surgical Conscience

- Surgical conscience requires the perioperative nurse to be engaged in continuous self-inspection coupled with the moral obligation to protect the patient.
- Surgical conscience consists of the following:
  - Adherence to standards from regulatory bodies
  - Commitment to high values, sense of duty, and ethical practice
  - Engaging in good personal hygiene and healthcare practices
  - Engaging in the correction of errors as soon as they are known (i.e., breaks in technique)
  - Establishing a rapport with the patient and family members
  - Maintaining accountability to the patient, employer, facility, profession of nursing, and the self
  - Monitoring of one's own professional behavior as well as others on the surgical team
  - Practicing in accordance with facility policy and standards of practice
  - Promotion of patient advocacy and attending to the needs of the family
  - Shared responsibility to ensure that the principles of asepsis and sterile technique are observed

Fostering a Culture of Safety

- A culture of safety is supported by the organization's leadership and encourages the following:
  - Acquiring appropriate resources and staff to safely complete the work
  - Avoidance of placing blame
  - Collaboration among all team members
  - Eliminating workplace violence (i.e., bullying, incivility, and horizontal or lateral violence)
  - Promotion of transparency, accountability, and teamwork
  - Trust among the members of the surgical team

THE INDIVIDUALIZED PLAN OF CARE

- The individualized plan of care is created at the time of the preoperative interview and is based on the type of surgery to be performed, the positioning needed to optimize the exposure of the surgical site, and specific needs associated with safety promotion.
- The perioperative nurse should develop an individualized plan of care that incorporates the use of the following:
  - Assessment data from the preoperative interview
  - Cultural sensitivity
  - NANDA guidance and diagnoses listing
  - Perioperative Patient Focused Model
  - PNDS
    - The nursing process (assessment, nursing diagnosis, planning, intervention, and evaluation)
- The nurse creates the individualized plan of care based on the type of surgery, which includes the following. Many of these categories can include the use of robotics.
  - *Cardiothoracic surgery:* Procedures that consist of repairs to the heart (i.e., coronary artery bypass graft)
  - *Craniotomy:* Procedures that focus on surgical intervention involving the brain or cranial bones
  - *General and gynecology:* Typically focused on the organs of the abdomen and pelvis

- *Endoscopy:* Procedures that use an endoscope and are focused on the alimentary canal
- *Neurosurgery:* Procedures that are focused on the nerves
- *Spinal surgery:* Procedures that focus on the repair of the vertebra and the spinal column
- *Ophthalmic surgery:* Procedures that focus on the repair of issues associated with the eyes
- *Organ procurement:* A procedure that is performed to procure organs for transplant and can consist of bone, eyes, and internal organs
- Orthopedic surgery and sports medicine:
  - *Orthopedic:* Procedures that consist of full or partial arthroplasty of the shoulder, hip, or knee
  - *Sports medicine:* Procedures that consist of repairs to ligaments, tendons, and soft tissue
- *Otorhinolaryngologic surgery (head and neck):* Procedures that consist of repairs to structures in the head, ears, or throat
  - Removal of organs is also performed through this type of surgery (e.g., thyroidectomy)
- *Plastic and reconstructive surgery:* Procedures that consist of repairs to any part of the body (e.g., breast augmentation or removal, facial reconstruction)
- *Urologic surgery:* Procedures that consist of repairs to the kidneys, bladder, ureters, penis, prostate, tumor removal, including vaginal reconstruction and stent placement
- *Vascular surgery:* Procedures performed to repair arteries or vasculature, or for stent or shunt placement
- The patient's positioning needs, the draping required, and the instrumentation to be used are specific to the type of procedure to be performed.
- The type of anesthesia to be administered depends solely on the judgment of the anesthesia team in collaboration with the surgeon and the patient.

Assessment Data

- Assessment data consists of the information collected from the preoperative interview and focused physical assessment.
- Individualizing the plan of care requires creating measurable patient outcomes based on assessment data and nursing diagnoses.
- Identify measurable patient outcomes throughout the perioperative phases: Preoperative, intraoperative, and postoperative. An example of an outcome statement for the individualized plan of care using the PNDS is "The patient will remain free from thermal injury."
- The perioperative nurse should use patient assessment data and nursing diagnoses to guide the selection of appropriate nursing interventions, establish a baseline for measuring the interventions' achievement, select a time frame to measure the achievement of the goal, and collect data based on its relationship to the surgical intervention.

 UNFOLDING SCENARIO 3A

Consider the following case study and the use of the nursing process.

A 20-year-old patient has been admitted directly to the presurgical holding area from the emergency department following a motor vehicle accident resulting in a head injury and a deep penetrating wound to the right leg. The patient is unconscious and unresponsive to noxious stimuli. The patient's mother confirms that the patient has no allergies or previous surgical history, is a nonsmoker, drinks on occasion, takes no medications, weighs 185 lb. and is 5 ft. 11 in. tall. The emergency department has removed all piercings. The surgeon states that the right leg will need to be amputated. Warm blankets are placed on the patient, and the patient is prepared for transport to the OR.

Question

What other aspects of the assessment are necessary?

Cultural Sensitivity

- The perioperative nurse should write culturally sensitive, age-appropriate, realistic, and measurable outcomes with interdisciplinary input, incorporating patient and family expectations.
- Ensure plan of care addresses patient-specific problems or considerations, including the following:
  - Age-specific considerations: Children and older adult patients require specific considerations related to positioning and normothermia.
  - Behavioral and physiologic reactions.
  - Community or social program accessibility: The patient's motivation to be proactive in postsurgical rehabilitation is influenced by access to care.
  - Cultural, ethnic, and religious impact on care:
    - Cultural differences will impact how the patient interacts with perioperative personnel and how they respond to treatment.
    - The patient's cultural influence will have an impact on the treatment they consent to be performed and how they interact with the surgical team. For example:
      - Consent for blood products may be impacted by religious beliefs.
      - Donation of organs may be prohibited by some cultures.
      - Eye contact may be prohibited by some cultures.
      - Some cultures require the provider to speak with the head of the family instead of the patient.
  - Disease processes implications:
    - Comorbid disease processes can create increased risks and postoperative complications. Examples are as follows:
      - COPD can affect the maintenance of anesthesia and intubation.
      - Congestive heart failure and history of heart disease affect circulation and hemodynamic stability.
  - Family pattern concerns and patient and family coping skills including suspected abuse.
  - Gender identification and history associated with gender transition therapy or surgery.
  - Ineffective family coping related to the surgical intervention, which can create preoperative anxiety for the patient and impact postoperative healing.

NANDA Guidance and Diagnoses

- NANDA diagnoses were developed in 1982 and are used to guide nurses and strengthen awareness related to the promotion of patient safety, improved patient outcomes, and quality of care.
- The four types of NANDA diagnoses and examples of each are presented in Table 3.1:

Table 3.1 NANDA Diagnoses		
NANDA Diagnosis	**Description**	**Example**
Health promotion	Goal to improve patient's overall health and well-being	Readiness for enhanced family coping related to surgical intervention
Problem-focused	Formulated during nursing assessment; chronic	Decreased cardiac output related to blood loss
Risk	Associated with development of a problem associated with the surgical intervention	Risk for imbalanced fluid volume related to blood loss
Syndrome	Associated with a pattern of issues related to the surgical intervention	Ineffective peripheral tissue perfusion related to blood loss

● Some of the most common NANDA nursing diagnoses for the perioperative setting are as follows. Table 3.2 details expected outcomes and appropriate nursing interventions for some of these diagnoses:
  ● Acute pain
  ● Anxiety
  ● Deficient knowledge
  ● Hyperthermia and hypothermia
  ● Ineffective airway clearance
  ● Ineffective coping
  ● Ineffective peripheral tissue perfusion
  ● Impaired gas exchange
  ● Impaired urinary elimination
  ● Readiness for enhanced comfort
  ● Risk for allergy reaction
  ● Risk for aspiration
  ● Risk for delayed surgical recovery
  ● Risk for electrolyte imbalance
  ● Risk for hypothermia
  ● Risk for imbalanced fluid volume
  ● Risk for impaired skin integrity
  ● Risk for infection
  ● Risk for injury
  ● Risk for perioperative positioning injury

POP QUIZ 3.1

Provide an example of a NANDA outcome statement related to electrical injury.

Table 3.2 Common Nursing Diagnoses for the Perioperative Patient

Nursing Diagnosis	Expected Outcome	Interventions
Anxiety	The patient will exhibit relaxed facial expressions and body movements.	● Address spiritual or cultural needs. ● Assess anxiety level. ● Explain the perioperative events. ● Greet the patient and ask how they would like to be addressed. ● Identify special concerns raised by the patient. ● Offer emotional support and reassurance.
Risk for SSI	The patient will remain free from infection.	● Adhere to usage instructions for all perioperative skin prep. ● Designate the appropriate wound classification. ● Identify patient-specific risk factors associated with maintaining hemodynamic stability skin integrity. ● Maintain patient normothermia throughout the procedure. ● Reduce traffic flow in the surgical suite. ● Review the patient history and physical. ● Use proper hand hygiene and aseptic technique. ● Verify the sterility of all items introduced to the sterile field. ● Verify that the room temperature is between 68 °F and 75 °F (20 °C–23.9°C) and humidity is between 20% and 60%.

(continued)

Table 3.2 Common Nursing Diagnoses for the Perioperative Patient *(continued)*

Nursing Diagnosis	Expected Outcome	Interventions
Risk for thermal injury	The patient will be free from thermal injury.	• Apply a grounding pad to protect the patient from electrical current. • Clean and dry skin prior to applying dressings. Remove all hair from the surgical site as indicated by the surgeon. • Preserve skin integrity. • Protect the patient from thermal, electrical, laser, and chemical injury in accordance with facility guidelines and manufacturer's instructions for equipment use. • Remove blood and body fluids from around the patient and apply a clean gown and blankets before transfer.
Risk for positioning injury	The patient will be free from signs and symptoms of positioning injury.	• Adjust the surgical table to meet the needs of the size of the patient. • Assess the patient for range of motion issues, prosthetics, and corrective devices. • Lift and transport the patient using the appropriate assistive equipment and personnel. • Reassess the patient for signs and symptoms of injury. • Use proper body alignment when positioning the patient and in consideration of limitations.
Risk for imbalanced fluid volume	The patient will maintain normal fluid volume during the surgical procedure.	• Assist anesthesia personnel with the collection of laboratory samples as needed. • Collaborate with the surgeon and anesthesia team on fluid replacement therapies. • Communicate blood loss through sponge count and suction container contents. • Review orders for blood and blood products and have them available or easily accessible prior to the procedure.
Risk for impaired tissue integrity	The patient's skin will remain intact.	• Apply dressings according to the surgeon's preferences to clean and dry skin. Assess the surgical incision for bleeding, drainage, and tissue integrity along the suture line. • Assess the surgical site for color, redness, swelling, warmth, and the patient's report of pain. • Assess other areas of the body for signs of skin integrity issues associated with pressure, friction, and shear.
Risk for hypothermia	The patient will retain an intraoperative core temperature of 96 °F–99 °F (35.6 °C–37.2 °C).	• Adjust the room temperature and humidity to accommodate for the preservation of normal body temperature. • Collaborate with the surgical team and anesthesia team related to the use of warmed IV fluid and warm sterile fluid dispensed to the surgical field. • Use warm blankets and forced-air warming devices to maintain normothermia.

UNFOLDING SCENARIO 3B

The patient has been transferred to the OR suite where the surgical team awaits. Bleeding has been controlled, and the patient's vital signs are stable. Upon moving the patient to the OR table, the nurse notices that there is a profuse amount of blood coming through the dressing on the right leg.

Question

What nursing diagnoses would be considered for this patient?

Using the PNDS for Outcome Identification

- The National Library of Medicine (2018) defines PNDS as a standardized nursing language used to support evidence-based perioperative nursing practice.
- PNDS is used to identify patient-specific diagnoses and select interventions for each to achieve expected outcomes including the following:
  - Nursing process framework
  - Patient-specific disease processes
  - Patient-specific nursing diagnoses
- PNDS has been integrated through AORN Syntegrity documentation to perform the following:
  - Assist in the measurement and evaluation of patient outcomes
  - Detect patient risks and associated evidence-based interventions
  - Identify deficiencies in documentation
  - Improve electronic documentation
  - Standardize documentation by providing a universal language
  - Support the creation of individualized patient-centered care plans
  - Support clinical practice

POP QUIZ 3.2

What are the four main purposes of PNDS in perioperative documentation?

UNFOLDING SCENARIO 3C

The patient is rapidly prepped and draped. The results of the CT scan of the head indicate that the patient has a concussion, and no cranial bleed is present. The surgeon begins the surgical assessment of the right leg. The circulating nurse calls for the time-out, and the team participates by pausing and confirming the right patient, site, procedure, equipment, and needs for the case.

Question

What should the nurse plan for next related to this case?

Perioperative Patient-Focused Model

- The Perioperative Patient Focused Model was developed by AORN and is an outcome-driven model used to describe the relationship between the perioperative nurse and the patient.
- There are four domains in this model:
  - Behavioral responses: Relate to the patient's behavioral response to perioperative care
  - Patient safety: Relates to the promotion of patient safety in the surgical environment
  - Physiologic responses: Relate to the patient's physiologic response to the surgical intervention
  - The health system: Relates to where the perioperative care is provided and the resources available
- The model aligns with the standards of perioperative nursing and addresses:
  - The responsibilities of the perioperative nurse who are associated with the role
  - The responsibility of each nurse to ensure that the work environment is safe and that adequate resources are available to provide care

(continued)

Perioperative Patient-Focused Model *(continued)*

- The requirement for the nurse to provide individualized care that is designed to meet unique patient needs, prevent injury, and encompass sensitivity to culture, race, ethnic diversity, and patient preference

The Nursing Process

- The perioperative nurse should document the ADPIE (common mnemonics are ADPIE and ANPIE).

 NURSING PEARL

Patient outcome statements are derived from the nursing diagnoses and formulated by collaborating with the patient, family members, and other members of the healthcare team.

- Assessment includes a review of the medical record, validation of important findings, collaboration with the patient, and accurate interpretation of clinical data.
  - The nursing diagnosis requires the synthesis of the data collected and the formulation of a clinical judgment.
  - Outcome identification in perioperative nursing is focused on preventative methods and generalized to all patients undergoing surgery.
  - Planning is associated with the formulation of nursing interventions to address the needs of the patient during all phases of perioperative care.
  - Evaluation is an ongoing process and incorporates the identification of outcomes that were met and those that will be communicated as needed to be met during handoff to the PACU.
- The documentation of patient care should include all aspects of the nursing process. The achievement of outcomes, as well as outcomes yet to be met, should be communicated to all members of the patient care team.
- The following nursing process components comprise the plan of care: Assessment, diagnosis, outcomes/planning, implementation, and evaluation.

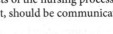 **NURSING PEARL**

Ida Jean Orlando-Pelletier introduced the well-known and universally used five stages of the deliberative nursing process theory that includes the following:

- Assessment
- Diagnosis
- Planning
- Implementation
- Evaluation

This process is sometimes called ADPIE.

  - Assessment
    - Analyze and prioritize pertinent findings.
    - Assess the patient's physical and psychosocial status.
    - Assess language and literacy skills.
    - Consider cultural and ethnic lifestyles.
    - Discuss elements around care with the patient as appropriate.
    - Review current diagnoses.
    - Review physiologic responses and psychosocial status.
    - Review previous hospitalizations or surgeries.
    - Review relevant components of the medical record.
    - Validate pertinent findings.
  - Diagnoses
    - Employ clinical reasoning and critical thinking skills to inform clinical judgment/diagnoses about the patient.
    - Include interventions that address the problem, signs, symptoms, etiology, and risk factors.
    - Synthesize data collected.
  - Outcome/planning
    - Include the patient and family in the formulation of the plan.
    - Incorporate knowledge of medical and surgical procedures.
    - Set nursing goals, establish desired outcomes, and plan interventions.
    - Use current best practices.

- Implementation
  - ○ Obtain all necessary supplies and equipment.
  - ○ Prepare the patient.
  - ○ Participate in patient transfer to the OR bed.
  - ○ Assist anesthesia personnel during intubation.
  - ○ Monitor for physiologic alterations.
  - ○ Perform the skin prep.
  - ○ Participate in draping the patient.
  - ○ Participate in the time-out.
  - ○ Participate in transfer from the OR to the next level of care.
  - ○ Provide a handoff communication to the receiving nurse.
- Evaluation
  - ○ Evaluate whether the patient is free from signs of injury.
  - ○ Determine whether the patient's vital signs are within normal limits.
  - ○ Use outcome statements for goals met or pending goals when providing a handoff.

UNFOLDING SCENARIO 3D

The amputation is complete, and the specimen is packaged for transport to pathology. The patient's vital signs remain stable, and no transfusion is needed. The surgeon and nurse first assistant begin primary closure of the wound. The scrub personnel begin to organize the instruments on the table.

Question

What is the nurse's next action?

UNFOLDING SCENARIO 3E

The surgical counts are completed and identified as correct. The dressings are applied, and a passive surgical drain is sutured into place by the surgeon. The nurse notices a pooling of prep solution under the thigh and blood on the gown.

Question

What is the nurse's next action?

RESOURCES

AORN Syntegrity. (2021). *Standardized nursing documentation with perioperative nursing data set (PNDS)*. https://www.aorn.org/syntegrity/products

Association for periOperative Registered Nurses. (2018). *PNDS (Perioperative nursing data set) – synopsis.* [Data set]. National Library of Medicine.

Association for periOperative Registered Nurses. (2019a). *Guideline essentials: Key takeaways.* [Poster/implementation tool]. https://www.aorn.org/essentials/information-management

Association for periOperative Registered Nurses. (2019b). *Is your periop documentation as optimized as it should be?* [Poster/PNDS decision support tool] https://www.aorn.org/syntegrity/resources

Association for periOperative Registered Nurses. (2021a). *2021 guidelines for perioperative practice.* Author.

Association for periOperative Registered Nurses. (2021b). *Environment of care (AORN guideline)*. https://aornguidelines.org/guidelines/content?sectionid=173720645&view=book#229132499

Nursing Theory. (n.d). *Ida Jean Orlando – Nursing theorist.* https://nursing-theory.org/nursing-theorists/Ida-Jean-Orlando.php

Phillips, N., & Hornacky, A. (2021). *Berry and Kohn's operating room technique* (14th ed.). Elsevier.

Rothrock, J. C., & McEwen, D. R. (2019). *Alexander's care of the patient in surgery.* Elsevier.

INTRAOPERATIVE PATIENT CARE AND SAFETY

OVERVIEW

- There are many interventions and actions needed for the perioperative nurse to complete in the intraoperative phase. In this chapter, the following topics are reviewed:
  - The time-out process
  - Patient positioning
  - Ergonomics and body mechanics
  - Anesthesia management
  - Surgical counts
  - Surgical site management
  - Management of equipment
  - Management of implants and explants
  - Intraoperative blood transfusion and salvage
- *Note:* Throughout each phase of the perioperative experience, the nurse will perform duties using the ACE process:
  - Assess
  - Confirm
  - Evaluate and Ensure

NURSE'S ROLE IN PATIENT CARE AND SAFETY

- The perioperative nurse serves many roles related to providing patient care and ensuring safety. These roles include patient advocate, observer, circulator, scrub, and manager of the surgical suite.
- The goal of perioperative nursing is to provide patients with a level of care that is collaborative, uses the most current evidence-based practice guidelines, enhances safety, is competent and makes use of critical thinking, and is patient centered.

Assess

1. Assessment of the perioperative patient is ongoing throughout the perioperative period and consists of the following:
   - Customizing care based on the patient's unique needs and the individualized needs of the procedure
   - Promoting physiological and psychological homeostasis
   - Providing privacy and dignity to the patient and their family members
   - Reducing stressful factors associated with the surgical environment
2. The primary function of the nurse related to continuous surgical field and intraoperative activity consists of the following:
   - Continuous assessment of the temperature and humidity in the surgical suite and reporting deviations from the facility and unit-based protocol

(continued)

Assess *(continued)*

- Evaluating procedure product and equipment packaging to ensure sterility parameters have been met
- Limiting staff movement within or outside of the sterile field to prevent the breach of sterility
- Performing equipment function testing to ensure functionality
- Reducing the risk of slip and fall and fire by performing an environmental scan

Confirm

1. Confirm that all patient safety needs have been addressed by the following:
   - Communicating to all levels of staff to ensure safety using standard handoff protocols
   - Disseminating and verifying the receipt of patient information
   - Developing and supporting a proactive approach to solving problems rather than a reactive and blaming approach
   - Encouraging a sense of trust among all team members through effective communication and adherence to policy and procedure
   - Having a commitment to affirming and making patient safety a priority

Evaluate and Ensure

1. The role of the perioperative nurse in promoting safety and providing patient care involves continuous evaluation of the following:
   - Environmental health hazards on and off the field
   - Equipment functionality
   - Location and placement of sharps, sponges, and other items that have the potential to be retained within a cavity
   - Patient's well-being during the continuum of care (e.g., blood loss, changes in vital signs, need for hemostatic agents)
   - Surgeon's needs and preferences for the case
2. The perioperative nurse also ensures that the following measures are taken to promote patient safety:
   - Ensures that the time-out process is performed
   - Limits the traffic and monitors movement in the three areas of the surgical unit:
     - *Unrestricted:* Outside the OR suites (PACU and waiting areas where street clothes may be worn)
     - *Semi-restricted:* OR holding area, scrub areas, and hallways around the surgical suites (where only scrub attire is permitted)
     - *Restricted:* OR suites and the sterile core or supply area (where masks and scrub attire are required)

TIME-OUT PROCESS

- The time-out process is the second phase of the Universal Protocol and is a team approach used to promote patient safety by ensuring the correct procedure is being performed on the correct patient.
- The purpose of the time-out is to prevent harm to the patient related to operating on the wrong site, operating on the wrong patient, or performing the wrong procedure.
- The time-out should occur after the patient has been prepped and draped for surgery and just before the surgical incision.

 ALERT!

The time-out process is one of the three phases of the Universal Protocol. The other aspects of the Universal Protocol, occurring before the patient is transported to the surgical suite, are conducting a preprocedure verification process and marking the procedural site. As of 2004, TJC identified that the Universal Protocol for Preventing Wrong Site, Wrong Procedure, Wrong Person Surgery is required for all accredited organizations.

UNFOLDING SCENARIO 4A

A 28-year-old patient has been transferred to the surgical suite for arthroscopic anterior cruciate ligament repair on the right knee. The patient is intubated, and a right femoral block is performed. The patient is positioned in the hemi-lithotomy position according to the surgeon's preference and is prepped and draped for surgery. The surgeon states that she is ready to begin.

Question

What should the perioperative nurse do next?

Assess

- Assess the activity in the room and ensure that all members of the surgical team are ready to conduct the time-out.
- If a patient has refused site marking or if site marking is impractical due to the nature of the surgery, adhere to the facility's policies and procedures.
- Examples of situations where marking may not be possible are as follows:
  - Dental surgery
  - Interventional procedures (i.e., cardiac catheterization, pacemaker insertion)
  - Surgery on infants, as the marking may leave a permanent stain on the skin
  - Surgery on mucosal surfaces, perineum, or internal organs (i.e., kidney, lung, ureter)

Confirm

- Confirm the following:
  - Designated person on the team begins the time-out process
  - Identity of the patient, the name of the procedure, incision site, presence of consent, and the visibility of the site marking
  - Involvement of all surgical team members
  - Use of a time-out for surgical cases where more than one surgery will be performed and when more than one surgeon is performing surgery
  - Use of a standardized process

Evaluate and Ensure

- Evaluate the activity in the room and ensure that the following activities occur:
  - A fire and safety risk assessment has been performed and confirmed with the surgeon.
  - All equipment needed for the procedure is available, and concerns have been verbalized.
  - Antibiotic prophylaxis has been administered within 1 hr of the initial surgical incision.
  - Relevant radiographic images are properly labeled and displayed where the team can see them.
  - Introduction of the surgical team members has been completed.
  - Surgical instrumentation to be used is confirmed as being sterile.
  - The patient has been positioned to maximize the exposure of the surgical site.
  - The surgeon has verbalized anticipated critical events (i.e., critical or nonroutine steps, a longer duration of the case, anticipated blood loss).
  - The sterilization indicators are present, viable, and visible, thus indicating that sterilization parameters have been met.

NURSING PEARL

I PASS CARE Mnemonic for Time-Out

- **I**ntroduce the team
- **P**rocedure
- **A**ssessment for fire and safety
- **S**ite confirmed and marked
- **S**terilization
- **C**onsent
- **A**ntibiotics administered
- **R**adiographs displayed
- **E**quipment available

UNFOLDING SCENARIO 4B

During the time-out process, the surgeon requests the x-rays and MRI image results.

Question

What should the perioperative nurse do?

PATIENT POSITIONING

- Patient positioning is a collaborative process that involves all surgical team members. The process consists of the following:
  - Thorough preoperative assessment
  - Selection of the appropriate equipment
  - Thorough postoperative evaluation of the patient after positioning is complete and before surgical draping
  - Documentation of the positioning process and materials used
- The goals of appropriate patient positioning are to perform the following:
  - Maintain the patient's privacy and comfort
  - Maximize surgical site exposure
  - Promote access to the IV lines for anesthesia and monitoring
  - Stabilize the patient to prevent friction and shear to the skin and patient shift during surgery
  - Maximize circulation and oxygenation
  - Promote perfusion to all vital organs and extremities
  - Protect the muscles, nerves, skin, joints, and vital organs from injury

Assess

1. Assess for potential positioning injuries related to the following:
   - Cold: Can reduce peripheral circulation, reduce oxygen delivery, and affect the skin and underlying tissue.
   - Heat: Can increase tissue metabolism, increase oxygen demand, and constrict or impede blood flow.
   - Moisture: Can macerate tissue causing the connective tissue to dissolve and tear. Moisture can present as patient perspiration, irrigants, blood, urine, fecal matter, or skin prep solution.
2. Assess surgical positioning for potential yet common positioning injuries, such as the following:
   - Stretching or compression of the brachial plexus, peroneal, and facial nerves:
     ○ The brachial plexus nerves are associated with compression or hyperflexion during positioning that involves the shoulder, hand, and arm.
     ○ The peroneal nerves are associated with compression during positioning that involves the leg, foot, and toes.
     ○ The facial nerves are associated with the positioning or compression of the face or areas of the neck.
3. During the assessment, consider the risks for positioning injuries, such as those with the following:
   - Bony prominences
   - External devices (e.g., catheters and colostomy bags)
   - High body mass index and obesity
   - Internally implanted devices (e.g., artificial joints and pacemakers)
   - Limited range of motion
   - Nutritional status
   - Preexisting conditions (e.g., peripheral vascular disease)
   - Presence or history of a pressure injury
   - Psychologic considerations (e.g., cognitively challenged)

- Skin tears, presence of rash, or history of skin breakdown
- Smoking, which causes vasoconstriction

4. Assess and select positioning equipment:
   - Select equipment based on surgeon preference list and special requests made by the surgeon.
   - Ensure all equipment and positioning aids are operational and intact and will not cause harm to the patient.
   - Inspect and maintain equipment on a regular basis and remove it from use if found nonoperational or damaged.

 NURSING PEARL

The pressure-relieving surface associated with positioning devices disperses the patient's body weight, alleviates pressure on bony prominences, and reduces pressure on the areas that are touching the OR table.

Confirm

- Confirm the appropriate positioning equipment is available based on the planned surgical positioning (Table 4.1).

Table 4.1 Common Patient Positions for Surgery

Position	Description	Positioning Equipment	Areas of Optimal Access

Supine	• The patient is lying flat on the back on the surgical table in an anatomic position.
	• Special attention should be placed on the position of the arms/hands.
	  ○ Palm up for traditional supine with arms extended
	  ○ Palms facing torso if tucked to side
	Note: If the arms are to be tucked for the procedure, use a sled positioner or be sure that there is a long enough draw sheet.
		• Bilateral arm boards (if required)
		• Foam or gel headrest
		• Gel pads
		• Foam or gel pad or blanket to elevate heels
		• Foam or gel knee positioner or blanket placed behind the knee to elevate the leg
		• Safety straps
			• Abdomen
			  ○ Abdominoplasty
			  ○ Appendectomy
			  ○ Cholecystectomy
			  ○ Laparoscopic abdominal procedures
			• Head
			  ○ Craniotomy
			  ○ Sinus surgery

Trendelenburg	• This is a commonly used position for abdominal surgeries that causes an elevation in cerebral blood and cerebrospinal fluid volume where the torso is lower than the legs.
	• The patient is lying on the back on the surgical table in an anatomic position.
	• The table is tilted with the head lower than the feet.
		• Bilateral arm boards (if required)
		• Foam or gel headrest
		• Gel pads
		• Foam or gel pad or blanket to elevate heels
		• Foam or gel knee positioner or blanket placed behind the knee to elevate the leg
		• Safety straps
			• Abdomen
			  ○ Colorectal surgery
			  ○ Gynecology procedures
			  ○ Laparoscopic abdominal procedures
			• Pelvis
			  ○ Robotic prostate surgery

(continued)

Table 4.1 Common Patient Positions for Surgery *(continued)*

Position	Description	Positioning Equipment	Areas of Optimal Access

Reverse Trendelenburg	• This is a position where the surgical site is elevated above the heart to improve drainage of fluids away from the site. This reduces intracranial pressure and improves pulmonary function where the torso is higher than the feet.
	• The patient is lying on the back on the surgical table in an anatomic position.
	• The table is tilted with the feet lower than the head.
		• Bilateral arm boards (if required)
		• Foam or gel headrest
		• Gel pads
		• Foam (or gel) pad or blanket to elevate heels
		• Foam or gel knee positioner or blanket placed behind the knee to elevate the leg
		• Padded footboard
		• Safety straps
			• Abdomen
			  • Bariatric surgery
			  • Laparoscopic abdominal procedures
			• Head and neck surgery

Sitting and modified sitting	• In this position, the patient is sitting with the head, neck, and torso elevated at 20° to 90°, the hips are flexed between 45° and 60°, and the knees flexed 30°.
	• The patient is in a sitting position. This position is also known as Fowler's, Semi-Fowler's, High-Fowler's, and beach chair.
		• Foam or gel headrest or padding to protect the occiput, scapulae, and ischial tuberosities
		• Foam or gel pads
		• Knee positioner to protect the back of the knees
		• Foam or gel pad under the ankles to elevate the heels
		• Footboard with foam or gel padding to prevent sliding and protect the feet
		• Safety straps
			• Chest
			  • Breast reduction
			• Head
			  • Nasal surgeries
			• Shoulder
			  • Shoulder arthroscopy and replacement

(continued)

Table 4.1 Common Patient Positions for Surgery *(continued)*

Position	Description	Positioning Equipment	Areas of Optimal Access

Lithotomy	• This position offers exposure to the vagina, rectum, and perineum through the use of stirrups for the legs. The upper body and torso are positioned flat on the surface of the OR table. There are five levels of lithotomy:
	 • Low: The patient's hips are flexed and lower legs are parallel with the OR table.
	 • Standard: The patient's hips are flexed at 80° to 100° and the lower legs are parallel with the OR table.
	 • Hemi: The patient's nonoperative leg is positioned in a supine and flat position while the operative leg is in traction or another positioning device (i.e., fracture table).
	 • High: The patient's hips are flexed and the stirrups are fully elevated.
	 • Exaggerated: The patient's hips are flexed and the lower legs are almost at a vertical position.
		• Foam or gel headrest
		 • Foam or gel pads
		 • Bilateral arm boards (if required)
		 • Padded stirrups to be positioned at the same height to avoid back strain and hip dislocation
		 • Candy cane stirrups may also be used (although not a current standard of practice)
		   • The patient's legs should be padded where the leg rests on the metal of the stirrup.
		 • Safety straps
			• Abdomen
			   • Colon surgery (low anterior colectomy)
			 • Pelvis
			   • Gynecology procedures
			   • Childbirth
			   • Hysterectomy
			   • Removal of bladder
			   • Urology procedures

Prone	• This position provides exposure to the sacral, rectal, or perineal areas and is also used for spinal procedures due to the reduction in abdominal pressure it affords.
	 • The patient is lying on the stomach.
		• Foam or gel headrest
		 • Foam or gel pads
		 • Foam or gel positioners, gel rolls, or blanket rolls (also known as chest rolls) under the shoulders, bilaterally
		 • Foam or gel knee pads
		 • Padded arm boards
		 • Foam or gel positioner under the ankles to elevate the feet
		 • Safety straps
			• Back
			   • Neurospine and cranial/brain surgery
			 • Extremities
			   • Surgery on the posterior aspect of the extremities
			 • Rectal surgery

(continued)

Table 4.1 Common Patient Positions for Surgery *(continued)*

Position	Description	Positioning Equipment	Areas of Optimal Access
Jackknife/Kraske	• The patient is lying on the stomach and the surgical table is lowered at the waist. The patient's head and feet are lower than the hips.	• Foam or gel headrest • Foam or gel pads • Foam or gel positioners or blanket rolls (also known as chest rolls) under the shoulders, bilaterally • Foam or gel knee pads • Padded arm boards • Foam or gel positioner under the ankles to elevate feet • Safety straps	• Pelvis • Rectal procedures

Lateral	• In this position, the patient is lying on the side. The dependent side, which is lying on the OR table, is the nonoperative side.	• Foam or gel headrest
		• Foam or gel pads
		• Foam or gel positioners under the arms
		• Axillary roll under the rib cage, posterior to the axilla
		• Upper arm on a padded arm board
		• Lower arm resting on a separate arm board
		• Pillow between the legs and padding for the ankles and feet
		• Safety straps
			• Abdomen
			  • Kidney surgery
			  • Liver surgery
			• Chest
			  • Lobectomy
			• Thorax
			  • Thoracotomy
			• Extremities
			  • Hip arthroplasty

Kidney	• The patient is lying on the side with the affected side up.
	• The kidney post is elevated once the patient has been positioned.
		• Foam or gel headrest
		• Foam or gel pads
		• Foam or gel positioners under the arms
		• Axillary roll under the rib cage, posterior to the axilla
		• Upper arm on a padded arm board
		• Lower arm resting on a separate arm board
		• Pillow between the legs and padding for the ankles and feet
		• Safety straps
			• Abdomen
			  • Kidney surgery
			  • Liver surgery
			• Chest
			  • Lobectomy
			• Thorax
			  • Thoracotomy

(continued)

Table 4.1 Common Patient Positions for Surgery *(continued)*

Position	Description	Positioning Equipment	Areas of Optimal Access

Fracture table	• The patient is lying flat on the surgical table from the lower back to the occiput. The arm on the operative side may be elevated in a sling or be secured across the chest (surgeon specific). The other arm is placed on a padded arm board or tucked. The nonoperative leg is placed in a padded leg holder. The operative leg is positioned in the traction boot.	• Foam or gel headrest
		• Foam or gel pads
		• Padded arm board
		• Extra padding for protection for all areas touching the bed
		• Safety straps
			• Lower extremities
			  ○ Hip fracture
			  ○ *Hip:* Intramedullary rod insertion
			  ○ Anterior hip arthroplasty

Knee–chest	• The patient can be lying lateral or prone. Prone and knee–chest position require additional padding for the knees and feet on a knee board.	• Foam or gel headrest
		• Foam or gel pads
		• Foam or gel positioners or blanket rolls (also known as chest rolls) under the shoulders, bilaterally
		• Foam or gel knee pads
		• Padded arm boards
		• Safety straps
			• Rectum
			  ○ Hemorrhoidectomy
			  ○ Pilonidal cyst removal

Wilson Frame	• A variation of the prone position to maximize exposure for spinal surgery. The chest and pelvis are elevated slightly.	• Foam or gel headrest
		• Foam or gel positioners or blanket rolls (also known as chest rolls) under the shoulders, bilaterally
		• Foam or gel knee pads
		• Padded arm boards
		• Foam or gel positioner under the ankles to elevate the feet
		• Safety straps
			• Back
			  ○ Neurospine surgery
			• Extremities
			  ○ Surgery on the posterior aspect of the extremities
			  ○ Rectal surgery
			• Rectum
			  ○ Hemorrhoidectomy
			  ○ Pilonidal cyst removal

Evaluate and Ensure

1. Evaluate the patient who is at higher risk for positioning complications, such as those who are obese:
   • Obese patients are at higher risk for airway compromise, difficult intubation, aspiration, hypoxia, cardiac issues, skin breakdown, and intraabdominal pressure.
   • Obese patients may require special equipment related to positioning, such as procedure beds that have a higher weight capacity, extra-long and wide safety straps, additional side-of-the-bed attachments, and additional positioning aids.

 ALERT!

A thorough assessment of the patient after positioning should be completed to evaluate and ensure that all risks for injury have been addressed.

(continued)

Evaluate and Ensure *(continued)*

2. Evaluate and ensure patients are protected from common positioning injuries, such as the following:
   - Cardiovascular
     - ○ Restriction to blood flow can lead to compromise, thrombosis, or stroke.
   - Eyes
     - ○ Improper position and lack of eye protection during surgery requiring the patient to be in the prone position for an extensive period of time can cause corneal abrasion and central retinal artery occlusion.
   - Internal organs
     - ○ Compression to the abdomen can cause hepatic dysfunction, abdominal compartment syndrome, venous congestion, and elevated intra-abdominal pressure that can decrease limb perfusion, cause tissue necrosis, and renal failure.
   - Nerves
     - ○ Stretching or compression can cause damage to the nerves with the most common sites of injury occurring at the brachial plexus, peroneal nerves, and facial nerves.
   - Lungs
     - ○ Poor positioning can cause reduced pulmonary functioning, such as hypoxia, decreased oxygen saturation, pulmonary edema, respiratory compromise, and atelectasis.
   - Skin
     - ○ Friction, pressure, and shearing can cause damage to the skin due to improper patient positioning.
       - ■ *Friction* is the force of two surfaces rubbing together.
       - ■ Pressure is associated with the force placed on the underlying tissue.
       - ■ Shearing is associated with the displacement of the skin from the underlying muscle.
3. Evaluate and ensure that the patient is protected from changes in temperature, moisture, and pressure.
   - Changes in temperature and heat exposure cause an increase in metabolism, which can impact blood loss, changes in anesthesia drug metabolism, and adverse cardiac events.
   - Excessive exposure to cold room temperatures or solutions can cause hypothermia.
   - Moisture can produce maceration of the skin and skin breakdown.
   - Pressure from wrinkles in the sheets, extra padding and linens, and additional layers can injure the skin.
4. Ensure the following occurs associated with protecting the patient from injury related to positioning:
   - Apply appropriate head support for the patient and avoid the use of towels or blankets that provide no cushion to the occiput.
   - Assess the patient's pulses before and after positioning.
   - Avoid extreme lateral rotation of the patient's head.
   - Avoid contact between the patient and the metal aspects of the OR table.
   - Collaborate with anesthesia personnel to ensure protection of the patient's airway at all times.
   - Continuously monitor the position of the patient's hands and fingers during all phases of positioning.
   - Do not allow equipment or heavy objects to rest on the patient.
   - Do not lean on the patient.
   - Do not allow the patient's extremities to fall below the level of the OR table.
   - Ensure that warming cabinet settings are consistent with the manufacturer's IFU to prevent fire and thermal injury to the patient.
   - Protect the patient's eyes with facility-approved eye protection or transparent dressings.

POP QUIZ 4.1

A 53-year-old female undergoes an elective total thyroidectomy for treatment of hypothyroidism. The patient is placed in the supine position with both arms tucked. What areas of the patient's body should the nurse pad to prevent injury?

UNFOLDING SCENARIO 4C

The patient undergoing a right knee arthroscopic anterior cruciate ligament repair is to be placed in the hemi-lithotomy position according to the surgeon's preference. The patient weighs 125 lb. and is 5 ft. 3 in. tall.

Question

What areas of the body should be padded?

ERGONOMICS AND BODY MECHANICS

Perioperative nurses need to utilize effective ergonomics and body mechanics while working in the surgical unit. The work performed in the surgical unit places a great degree of stress and strain on the body. By ensuring that appropriate ergonomic tools are used, the nurse promotes safety in the work environment.

Assess

1. Assess the following pertaining to the surgical procedure:
- Access to transfer devices
- Assistive personnel needed to safely transfer the patient to and from the stretcher to the OR table
- Equipment to be moved for the procedure
- Height and weight of the patient
- Patient's range of motion and ability to move independently
- Patient's risk for fall
- Surgical position to be used for the procedure and associated positioning equipment needs

2. Assess the high-risk tasks involved with performing the procedure, such as the following:
- Patient transfer and positioning
- Holding retraction
- Movement of equipment

Confirm

1. Confirm the following related to the use of appropriate body mechanics:
- All staff are using ergonomic tools to move patients safely.
- Effective communication is used to evaluate and ensure safe patient movement and reduce the risk of injury to staff members.

2. Confirm that risk-reduction strategies have been considered, such as the following:
- Conduct an ergonomic assessment of the suite and overall work environment.
- Participate in risk-reduction and quality improvement activities.
- Request assistance when lifting a heavy load or heavy equipment.
- Report ergonomic and work environment safety hazards to supervisors.

Evaluate and Ensure

1. Evaluate the physical stressors associated with patient or equipment movement, such as the following:
- Awkward and static postures, which are associated with holding the patient, are steady for prepping and draping
- Forceful exertion or overexertion, which is associated with the transfer of heavy equipment
- Lifting or carrying heavy patients or equipment and instrumentation
- Long work hours

(continued)

Evaluate and Ensure *(continued)*

- Prolonged standing
- Repetitive motions

2. Evaluate that the fundamentals of patient transfer are observed by all staff members and include the following considerations:
   - Can the patient transfer without assistance?
   - How many staff members are needed?
   - What is the starting position?
   - What is the final position?
   - What is the patient's weight?
   - What devices are needed?

3. Ensure the following actions are considered to reduce risks associated with excessive standing:
   - Adjust the height of the OR table.
   - Alternate sitting and standing when possible.
   - Prop feet on a stool if the procedure requires standing for more than 2 hr
   - Use antifatigue mats where feasible.
   - Wear supportive footwear that does not change the shape of the foot, is spacious enough inside to move toes, and is shock absorbent.

4. Ensure the following steps are considered when performing patient transfers:
   - Proper body alignment is maintained.
   - Provide support to the patient's extremities and airway.
   - The number of personnel is adequate to safely transfer the patient.
   - Use assistive devices to facilitate patient transfer from one surface to another.
   - Work as a team to reduce the risk of injury to all personnel.

 ALERT!

According to AORN's 2021 guidelines for safe patient handling and movement, high-risk perioperative nursing tasks are patient transfers, repositioning of patients, lifting, and holding extremities, standing, holding retractors, lifting and moving equipment, and sustaining awkward positions for extended periods of time.

 UNFOLDING SCENARIO 4D

The surgery on the patient undergoing the right knee arthroscopic anterior cruciate ligament repair has been completed, and it is time to move the patient back to the supine position.

Question

What considerations should the nurse make when repositioning the patient?

ASSISTING WITH ANESTHESIA MANAGEMENT

The perioperative nurse assists the anesthesia personnel from the point of induction to extubation.

Assess

1. Assess the following associated with the planned procedure:
   - Length of surgery
   - Patient age
   - Physiologic status of the patient

2. Assess the planned position for the procedure:
   - Postoperative recovery time
   - Previous experience and history with anesthesia

- Surgery planned
- Type of anesthesia to be administered
3. Assess the following stages of anesthesia during the procedure:
    - Stage 1: Analgesia or disorientation
        - This stage is marked by sedation with conversation that lasts from the time of initial administration of anesthesia to the loss of consciousness.
    - Stage 2: Excitement or delirium
        - This stage is marked by features such as disinhibition and delirium and lasts from the time of loss of consciousness to the loss of eyelid reflex.
    - Stage 3: Surgical anesthesia
        - At this time, the patient is fully sedated under surgical anesthesia.
    - Stage 4: Respiratory arrest
        - This stage is a state of respiratory failure leading to circulatory failure and death.
4. Assess the following phases of anesthesia:
    - Induction: This phase begins with the administration of anesthesia and lasts until the surgical incision.
    - Maintenance: This phase occurs after the surgical incision and lasts until near completion.
    - Emergence: This phase begins as the patient awakens.

Confirm

1. Confirm the patient's ASA score with the anesthesia provider:
    - ASA I: Normal and healthy patient
    - ASA II: Patient with mild systemic disease (smoker, social drinker, pregnancy, controlled diabetes, hypertension, mild lung disease, obesity)
    - ASA III: Patient with severe systemic disease (DM, hypertension, morbid obesity, COPD)
    - ASA IV: Patient with severe systemic disease that is a constant threat to life (myocardial infarction, cerebrovascular attack, trans-ischemic attack within 3 months)
    - ASA V: Moribund patient who is not expected to survive without the surgery or operation (ruptured abdominal aortic aneurysm, thoracic aneurysm, massive trauma, intracranial bleed, ischemic bowel)
    - ASA VI: Patient who has been declared brain-dead and whose organs are being donated

Evaluate and Ensure

1. Ensure that the perioperative nurse is working within the scope of practice outlined in their state's nurse practice acts when asked to assist the anesthesia provider.
2. Evaluate and ensure that the perioperative nurse supports the patient at the bedside.
3. Evaluate the needs of the anesthesia staff during general anesthesia, local anesthesia, regional anesthesia, and moderate sedation/analgesia.

> **◢))) ALERT!**
>
> The perioperative nurse should work within the scope of practice and cannot fulfill the dual roles of the circulator and local/moderate sedation monitoring nurse.

- General anesthesia: The perioperative nurse provides ancillary assistance to, and works under the guidance of, the anesthesia team during induction and emergence. The perioperative nurse may be required to apply cricoid pressure during intubation and serves as a support for the patient.
- Local anesthesia: The perioperative nurse may be required to provide patient monitoring during the administration of local anesthesia through the following interventions:
    - Application of monitoring devices (blood pressure cuff, pulse oximetry, electrocardiogram)
    - Evaluation and documentation of vital signs
    - Positioning of the patient to ensure maximum exposure for surgery and comfort while in position

(continued)

Evaluate and Ensure *(continued)*

- Moderate sedation/analgesia: The perioperative nurse may be required to administer medications and assess vital signs at prescribed intervals during the procedure.
- Regional anesthesia: The perioperative nurse may be required to assist during regional anesthesia through the following:
  - Assessment of the type of medication used
  - Assisting with the placement of monitoring devices
  - Evaluation and assessment of vital signs
  - Supporting the patient during positioning (i.e., spinal placement)

4. Evaluate the needs of the anesthesia personnel related to patient reactions and the risks associated with anesthesia such as the following:
   - Bradycardia
   - Fever
   - Hematoma
   - Hypotension
   - LAST
   - Nausea and vomiting
   - Postdural puncture headache
   - Pruritus
   - Shivering
   - Urinary retention

5. Ensure the following nursing interventions are provided during the course of the procedure:
   - Ensure the safety of the environment
   - Comfort patient
   - Set up equipment and obtain blood products, if needed
   - Maintain the integrity of the sterile field
   - Assist by initiating the flow of IV, if clamped off
   - Facilitate intubation by holding for cricoid pressure (general anesthesia)
   - Assist with induction and emergence (general anesthesia or moderate sedation)
   - Assist with suction
   - Ensure safe handling and dispensation of medications and sharps during the course of the procedure and to the sterile field

 ALERT!

The perioperative nurse should review the plan for anesthesia with the anesthesia team and the surgeon related to the medications to be used, the route of administration, the length of the procedure, and other risk-related concerns.

NURSING PEARL

Surgical patients have significant anxiety when entering the surgical suite; therefore, the perioperative nurse plays an important role in reducing this anxiety and assisting the anesthesia staff to deliver safe effective care.

SURGICAL COUNTS

- The unintended retention of foreign objects remains the top-reported sentinel event through TJC.
- Ensuring counts of surgical items at risk for retention based on the procedure are completed reduces the risk of foreign object retention in the patient.

Assess

Assess the surgical field and perform the surgical count as follows (based on the surgical procedure):

- Before the start of the surgical procedure
- Upon dispensing sharps, sponges, or instrumentation to the surgical field
- Upon closing a cavity within a cavity
- Upon closing the first layer (e.g., fascia)
- Upon final closure
- When permanent relief of either a scrub person or nurse circulator occurs

 ALERT!

There may be exceptions to instrument counting per facility policy.

Confirm

1. Confirm the count between the scrub person and nurse circulator. If a counting error exists, perform the following:
   - Identify errors in counting immediately and report them to the surgeon.
   - Stop all activity and begin a recount.
   - Follow facility policy associated with counts that cannot be reconciled.
2. Confirm that the instruments and devices are intact when they are returned to the field from the operative site.
3. Verify the integrity and completeness of all items when counting.

Evaluate and Ensure

1. Evaluate the surgical site and remove all soft goods, instruments, and sharps before counting. Key items to remember are as follows:
   - Do not use towels inside the wound.
   - Sponges should be radiopaque.
   - When the wound is intentionally packed with radiopaque or nonradiopaque sponges, document the count once confirmed with the surgeon and communicate the number of retained sponges to the receiving unit.
2. Ensure that counts are not being performed during critical times during a procedure.
   - *Note:* Anyone can call for an additional count at any time during the procedure. The surgeon has the authority to override the decision to perform a count during critical times. Adherence to hospital policy must be maintained.
3. Ensure that the circulating nurse can visibly see all items during the count.

> **ALERT!**
>
> Both the circulator and scrub must be able to visualize all items during the count. Do not count product packages. The nurse circulator and the scrub person must count all physical soft goods, sharps, and instruments.

STERILE FIELD MANAGEMENT

The principles of aseptic technique are associated with using all items that have been appropriately sterilized, stored in sterile areas, and only come into contact with persons who are authorized to handle sterile.

Assess

Assess the following associated with maintaining sterility:
- All items for use in the procedure must be sterile.
- Assess the integrity of all items dispensed to the surgical field.
- Compromised barriers are considered contaminated.
- Draped tables are sterile only at the table level or top surface.
- Edges of a sterile wrapper or container are considered unsterile.

Confirm

1. Confirm that only persons considered sterile are touching the sterile field.
   - Gowns have established parameters of sterility:
     - Once donned, sleeves are sterile up to 2 in. above the elbows.
     - The front of gown is sterile from chest to level of the sterile field.
     - The back of the gown is not considered sterile.
   - Restrict movement around the sterile field.
2. Confirm that the donning of gloves and gowns adheres to AORN recommendations and facility policy:
   - Hand hygiene is performed.
   - Inspection of the integrity of the gown and gloves has been performed.

(continued)

Confirm (*continued*)

- Removal of contaminated gloves or gown is done promptly.
- Selection of the surgical gown is associated with the degree of exposure.
- Sterile technique is followed when donning the gown and gloves.

Evaluate and Ensure

1. Evaluate the movement of all personnel in and around the sterile field.
2. Evaluate the following associated with the preparation of the sterile field:
   - Do not move the sterile field beyond the surgical suite where it was originally opened.
   - Prepare the sterile field as close to the time of actual use as possible.
   - Only sterile items should come into contact with the sterile field.
   - Use an isolation technique when working in a procedure involving the bowel, resection of metastatic tumors, or infected tissue.
3. Ensure the following protocol is maintained throughout the procedure:
   - Limit traffic in the surgical suite and keep the OR suite doors shut.
   - Limit exposure of the other materials in the sterile field when hydrotherapy or debridement with irrigation is occurring.
   - Monitor for breaks in sterility.
   - Open and deliver sterile items in a manner that serves to maintain sterility.
   - Open the sterile items according to the manufacturer's IFU.
   - Review and follow the facility's policy if case is delayed and follow the procedure for covering the field or portions of the field when not in use.
   - Sterile persons must pass each other face-to-face or back-to-back and keep their lower arms up above the waist.
   - Unsterile persons should not walk between areas of sterility.
4. Ensure the scrubbed members of the surgical team do the following throughout the procedure:
   - Avoid changing levels of the hands, table height, or OR table height.
   - Avoid turning the back on the sterile field.
   - Avoid folding of the arms, as no part of the hands or arms should be under the axilla.
   - Remain close to the sterile field.
   - Keep hands and arms above waist level.
   - Use shielding devices when radiologic exposure is expected.

NURSING PEARL

When in doubt, throw it out! Any member of the surgical team can determine that there is a contamination. The more eyes on the sterile field and around the sterile field, the better. If there is uncertainty about any item, the intraoperative nurse should discard the disposable item or return the instrumentation to sterile processing in accordance with facility policy and procedure.

POP QUIZ 4.2

The scrub nurse performs a check of sharps during a carotid endarterectomy. The scrub alerts the circulating nurse and the surgeon that one of the vascular needles is missing. The surgeon states that this is a critical point in the procedure, and he cannot stop to do a full count. What is the circulating and scrub nurse's next action?

SURGICAL SITE MANAGEMENT

The perioperative nurse must work to reduce the risk of surgical site exposure to infectious materials.

Assess

1. The circulating nurse and scrub person must continually assess the surgical site and area surrounding it to ensure that foreign bodies are not lost within a cavity or wound.
2. Assessment activities include the following:
   - Assessing the integrity of gloves and gowns worn by those at the surgical field
   - Confining and containing spills to protect the integrity of the field and the tables
   - Continuous evaluation of the integrity of surgical drapes
   - Monitoring for breaks in technique

Confirm

Confirm all actions within the sterile field adhere to aseptic technique and work to maintain the sterility of the field, such as the following:

- Only scrubbed personnel should move within the sterile field.
- Sterile draping should cover all areas designated as the sterile field.
- Items used within the sterile field should be inspected first (expiration dates, sterilization indicators), then presented to the sterile field.
- Delivery of all items to the sterile field, including medications, should be performed using an aseptic technique.
- Traffic around the sterile field and within the surgical suite should be limited.

Evaluate and Ensure

1. Evaluate the integrity of the following:
   - Gowns and drapes
   - Sterile supply packaging
   - Sterilization through the presence of external and internal sterilization indicators
   - Rigid container seals and locks
2. Ensure that the surgical wound is kept clean and free from packages, nonradiopaque sponges, and items not immediately used for the particular phase of surgery.

ALERT!

Foreign bodies left inside a patient's wound create serious harm. The surgical team should ensure that proactive risk strategies are used to prevent the occurrence of retained surgical items and work to reduce the risk for infection at the surgical site by maintaining the sterility of the field.

PERSONAL PROTECTIVE EQUIPMENT

The PPE and surgical attire worn in the OR should ensure a high level of cleanliness and hygiene, reduce the patient's exposure to microorganisms, reduce the risk for SSI, and protect staff from cross contamination.

Assess

ALERT!

Effective in July 2019, these guidelines for surgical attire were approved by the AORN Guidelines Advisory Board.

1. Assess the integrity of surgical scrubs and ensure that only those that are laundered through the healthcare facility's approved site are used.
2. Assess that all members of staff at the surgical field wear appropriate PPE such as eyewear, masks, and clean gowns.
3. Ensure that gowns that are penetrated with blood or have experienced strikethrough from sharps are removed.

Confirm

1. Confirm that the scrub attire is
   - clean,
   - covering areas of the body that shed (hair, arms, beard),
   - nonlinting,
   - safe for use (foot protection and shoes should adhere to OSHA regulations and American Society for Testing and Materials (ASTM) F2414 standards), and
   - stored in enclosed carts or containers and in a manner that prevents contamination.
2. Confirm that PPE is
   - fluid resistant (surgical gowns, gloves, and cover apparel),
   - cleaned between cases if not disposable (specialty eye protection), and
   - discarded after the case if disposable.

Evaluate and Ensure

1. Evaluate the field for strikethrough and torn gloves.
2. Ensure that breaks to the integrity of PPE are addressed promptly.
3. Ensure staff is protected from cross contamination.

ENVIRONMENTAL MANAGEMENT IN THE SURGICAL SUITE

Environmental management in the surgical suite includes the following:

- Chemical management (methyl methacrylate, glutaraldehyde, formaldehyde, formalin)
- Environmental cleaning
- Fire prevention
- Noise control and reduction
- Surgical smoke
- Thermal injury reduction

Assess

Assessment of the surgical environment is continuous and should address the following key areas related to the environment of care:

- Chemical management on and off the field
- Fire prevention and protection of patient from injury
- Level of noise occurring within the surgical suite
- Environmental cleaning to reduce the risk of infection
- Thermal injury reduction to the patient and staff

Confirm

Confirm the following are addressed:

- Chemical management on and off the field
  - An MSDS should be available for all chemicals.
  - Appropriate PPE (masks, gloves, and eyewear) should be worn when handling chemicals.
  - Chemicals are stored in an area that is well ventilated and according to federal, state, and local regulations.
- Environmental cleaning
  - Cleaning should occur between each surgical case.
  - Do not use spray bottles or brooms, as contamination can be spread through these methods.
  - Environmental service personnel should follow surgical attire guidelines.
  - Floors should be mopped with damp or wet mops.
  - Selection of products should be done using a chemical hazard assessment.
  - Terminal cleaning should occur at the end of the day.
  - Use designated cleaning equipment.
- Fire prevention
  - Assess the type of skin prep used (is it flammable?).
  - Assess types of ignition and fuel sources present (anesthesia gases, gases used in surgery, fluids used in surgery, electrocautery, drapes, gowns, the patient).
  - Check testing of lasers or fiberoptic lighting and the spatial relationship to the drapes.
  - Check the potential for the presence of high oxygen levels.
  - Ensure that instruments and equipment to be used (electrocautery, heated probes, defibrillators, drills, saws, burrs) are not lying on the drapes.

 POP QUIZ 4.3

The scrub person is setting up the sterile field for an abdominal aortic aneurism procedure. As the circulating nurse requests to begin the surgical count, she notices that there is strikethrough on the scrub person's gown. What is the circulating nurse's next action?

NURSING PEARL

The fire triangle consists of the ignition source, the oxidizer, and the fuel source.

 ALERT!

Surgical fires can occur at any location in the fire triangle. The perioperative nurse must know how to extinguish a fire and evacuate the OR and surgical suite.

- Noise control and reduction
  - Control the tone of conversations and extraneous distracting noise.
  - Limit conversations that are not essential to the case.
  - Limit the traffic within the surgical suite and the number of times the door is opened.
  - Limit the use of communication devices, phones, and wireless systems.
  - Reduce extraneous noise from music and equipment where feasible.
- Surgical smoke management
  - Evacuation of surgical smoke is performed by the surgical team.
  - The smoke evacuation system is functioning and has a clean filter in place.
  - PPE is worn when disposing of the filter.
  - Wall suction should be operational and verified at the surgical field.
- Thermal injury reduction
  - Control the temperature of fluids used in the procedure.
  - Implement a maximum temperature limit for blanket warming cabinets based on manufacturer guidelines.
  - Monitor the placement of electrocautery instrumentation, fiberoptic cables, and laser equipment at the sterile field.

Evaluate and Ensure

1. Evaluate that all safety measures are followed pertaining to facility policies and procedures.
2. Ensure the following related to surgical skin prep and fire safety:
   - Allow flammable skin antiseptics to dry completely and fumes to dissipate before surgical drapes are applied and before using a potential ignition source (e.g., ESU, laser).
   - Allow flammable solutions (e.g., alcohol, collodion, tinctures) to dry completely and fumes to dissipate before using an ignition source.
   - Conduct a skin prep time-out to validate that the skin antiseptic is dry before draping the patient.
   - Conduct, document, and communicate the completion of the fire risk assessment.
   - Remove materials that are saturated with the skin antiseptic agent before draping the patient.
   - Use reusable or disposable sterile towels to absorb drips and excess solution during application.
   - Wick excess solution with a sterile towel to help dry the surgical prep area completely.

 POP QUIZ 4.4

A 42-year-old female underwent a radical hysterectomy and sentinel node biopsy. The surgeon accidentally activates the monopolar current that was lying on the drape instead of the bipolar forceps. The foot pedals are pushed under the surgical table. A spark ignites the drape. What is the circulating nurse's first course of action?

MANAGEMENT OF EQUIPMENT AND MATERIALS

The perioperative nurse and surgical staff should use all equipment and surgical materials according to the manufacturer's recommendations.

Assess

Assess the function of all equipment to be used in a surgical case on and off the field.

Confirm

1. Confirm that the special equipment to be used is available and functional.
2. Confirm that required equipment has been tested preoperatively as appropriate.

Evaluate and Ensure

1. Evaluate equipment, ensure its function, and examine for fire hazards:
   - Electrosurgery
     - *Capacitive coupling:* A natural radio frequency phenomenon that can occur when energy is transferred through intact insulation on the shaft of a laparoscopic instrument to a nearby conductive material
     - *Direct coupling:* Occurs when the active electrode accidentally touches another noninsulated metal instrument allowing electrical energy to flow from one to the other
     - *Insulation failure:* Occurs when the insulation coating of an endoscopic instrument has been compromised
   - Lasers
     - All personnel in the room should wear eyeglasses/safety goggles designed for laser safety specific to the type of laser being used. There are three main types of laser beams:
       - *Collimated:* Waves parallel to each other that do not diverge significantly.
       - *Coherent:* All the waves are orderly and in phase with each other as they travel in the same direction.
       - *Monochromatic:* Photons with the same wavelength and color.
     - There are many safety issues to be reviewed related to lasers and human tissue, such as the following:
       - *Absorption safety:* Laser beam can produce a photothermal effect and burn the tissue it touches.
       - *Reflection safety:* Ensure laser does not inadvertently strike untargeted areas.
       - *Scattering safety:* Ensure laser light beam does not backscatter and cause damage to the scope, the optics, or the operator's eye.
       - *Transmission safety:* Ensure argon beam is not transmitted through fluid and structures of the eye to the retina, causing thermal photocoagulation.

ALERT!

Laser Safety
- The laser must display a warning label, per federal regulation.
- The laser aperture through which the laser beam is emitted must be clearly marked.
- When a laser filter is used in the microscope, the filter placement must be checked by two people, at least one of whom is a RN.
- The laser operator will be knowledgeable of and accountable for all laser safety in accordance with manufacturer instructions and facility policy and procedure.

   - Pneumatic tourniquets
     - Ensure the following steps are followed:
       - Choose the optimal location.
       - Follow the manufacturer's instructions.
       - Use natural rubber latex tourniquets, if indicated.
       - Use a physical barrier.
       - Verify the surgical site.
   - Ultrasonic instruments
     - *Ultrasonic instruments* are vibrating devices that deliver high-frequency sound waves transmitted down the shaft to the tip of the instrument to cut or coagulate.
     - Mechanical motion causes the tissue protein to become denatured as the hydrogen bonds are broken.
     - Ensure that all cords and cables are covered in a protective sheath.
2. Ensure that the surgical suite is made ready for the patient by the following processes:
   - Checking that the suite has IV poles and related equipment
   - Collecting all intraoperative medications and dispensing them to the field using aseptic technique
   - Dispensing supplies to the sterile field aseptically
   - Leveling the surgical table and gathering all positioning equipment
   - Selecting and examining sterile supplies according to the physician preference list
   - Testing the suction and making sure suction equipment is available

MANAGEMENT OF IMPLANTS AND EXPLANTS

- Implants and explants should be handled using aseptic technique.
- Some devices require tracking. Facility policy and procedure manuals should outline the process of tracking, reporting, handling, returning, submitting to pathology, documenting, and disposing, as well as protocols on returning to patients.

Assess

1. Assess the packaging of all implantable material before dispensing it to the surgical field.
2. Assess the requirements for handling of explants related to final disposition.

Confirm

1. Confirm with the surgeon the implant to be dispensed to the field.
   - Autologous tissue management consists of the following:
     - Facilities may be registered with the U.S. FDA as a tissue establishment, commonly referred to as a tissue bank. Facilities registered as tissue establishments must meet the laws outlined in the Code of Federal Regulations Chapter 21, Part 1271.
     - In some states, tissue banks must be also licensed in that particular state and registered with the AATB.
2. Confirm the explant identification with the surgeon.

Evaluate and Ensure

1. Evaluate the special handling protocols of the implant according to the manufacturer's recommendations.
2. Ensure that the information on the implant has been recorded for tissue tracking purposes, if applicable.
3. Evaluate the following related to the handling of explants:
   - Chain of custody (e.g., forensic evidence)
   - Device failure and return to the manufacturer
   - Tissue tracking

 ALERT!

There are times when law enforcement is waiting for evidence (e.g., knife fragments, bullet fragments). Adhere to facility policy and requirements of the law enforcement agency when handling these items.

INTRAOPERATIVE BLOOD TRANSFUSION AND SALVAGE

The intraoperative nurse should assess the need for blood salvage and blood products related to the surgical procedure.

Assess

1. Assess for adverse effects associated with surgical bleeding, such as the following:
   - Blood loss requiring blood transfusion
   - Reduction in core body temperature
   - Hypovolemic shock
   - Thrombocytopenia
   - Visual obstruction at the surgical field
2. Assess the patient for the following issues associated with the use of hemostatic agents:
   - Allergies to any topical hemostatic agent or products of bovine or porcine origin
   - Personal or family history of bleeding disorders, bleeding gums, easy bruising, excessive superficial bleeding, severe nosebleeds, anemia, or renal or hepatic disease
   - Use of anticoagulants or anti-PLT medications

(continued)

Assess *(continued)*

- Use of aspirin-containing or other nonsteroidal antiinflammatory prescription or over-the-counter medication
- Use of supplements or herbs that might contribute to increased bleeding times
3. Assess the following related to the need for blood products using the TAPE mnemonic:
   - Type of procedure
   - Anticipated blood loss
   - Presence of type and cross match in the patient's lab results
   - Evaluation provided by the surgeon

Confirm

1. Confirm the patient's medication history related to the use of anticoagulants.
2. Confirm the need for blood products with anesthesia personnel and the surgeon.

Evaluate and Ensure

1. Evaluate the need for blood products and blood salvage. The objectives of transfusion are to perform the following:
   - Increase circulating blood volume after surgery, trauma, or hemorrhage.
   - Increase the number of circulating RBCs and maintain HGB levels in patients with anemia.
   - Provide selected cellular components as replacement therapy.
2. Evaluate the factors that contribute to surgical bleeding, such as the following:
   - Patient factors
     - Anatomic anomalies
     - Coagulopathies and comorbidities
     - Medications
     - Nutritional status
   - Procedural factors
     - Dissection of adhesions
     - Exposed capillaries
     - Exposure of bone
     - Friable tissue
     - Patient positioning
     - Type of procedure
     - Type of surgical incision to be made
     - Unseen or unexpected sources of bleeding
3. Ensure that the requirements for blood transfusion are met:
   - Blood checked by two RNs or per institution policy
   - Patient consent obtained
   - Large gauge IV (#20 smallest) availability
   - Patient response to transfusion (e.g., transfusion reactions and fluid volume excess)
   - Physician's order
   - Vital signs to be taken as per institution policy
   - Secondary IV line with normal saline only
4. Ensure that assistance is provided to the surgeon to promote safe surgical hemostasis and reduce the risk for the need for infusion through the use of the following:
   - Mechanical methods
     - Direct pressure
     - Sponges
     - Sutures, staples, ligation clips
   - Pharmacologic agents
     - Desmopressin
     - Epinephrine

- ○ Lysine analogues
- ○ Protamine
- ○ Vitamin K
- Thermal- and energy-based methods
  - ○ Electrosurgery through the use of monopolar, bipolar, and argon-enhanced coagulation
  - ○ Laser
  - ○ Ultrasonic devices
- Topical hemostatic agents
  - ○ Cellulose
  - ○ Collagen-based products
  - ○ Gelatin
  - ○ Polysaccharide spheres
  - ○ Sealants such as fibrin
  - ○ Thrombin products

 ALERT!

- Transfusion reactions can happen immediately. Be vigilant in assessing the patient's vital signs post transfusion.
- The use of hemostatic agents (topical and pharmacologic) is contraindicated for use during cell salvage.

SPECIMEN MANAGEMENT

- A specimen is any blood, soft tissue, bone, body fluid, or foreign body that has been ordered by the surgeon to be sent to the pathology lab for analysis.
- AORN recommends that the transfer of all specimens from the sterile field occur as soon as possible using sterile technique and standard precautions.
- AORN recommends that the integrity of the specimen is preserved during transfer.

Assess

1. Assessment of specimen collection and special handling needs should begin when the procedure is scheduled.
2. Assess that the process of specimen collection aligns with facility policy and incorporates the following:
   - Dedicated specimen collection process and transfer system
   - Reduction in the number of people involved in the process
   - Standardized process

Confirm

Confirm the following are completed related to specimen management:
- Breast cancer specimen handling should be streamlined and include the following related to documentation and disposition:
  - Time of excision and fixation (if required)
  - Transfer to pathology as soon as possible and record the time of transfer
  - Use of radiologic imaging (if needed)
- Collection and handling of a specimen should be maintained in a manner that prevents misidentification or mishandling.
  - Documentation and labeling should include the following:
    - ○ Type of specimen and patient information (name, age, history, diagnosis)
    - ○ Study required, date and time of collection, and information pertinent to the specimen
    - ○ Surgeon's name and responsible party's signature

 ALERT!

Specimen Containment Guidelines
- If one specimen container is compromised, it must be placed in a second leak-proof container.
- If the exterior surface of a container is considered contaminated during handling, it should be placed into a specimen bag.

(continued)

Confirm *(continued)*

- Patient and specimen identification should be made just before the removal of the specimen from the surgical field.
- Specimen containers should be labeled to communicate patient, specimen, preservative, and biohazard information.
- Tissue specimens should be designated for a routine pathologic exam, gross identification only, or disposal according to healthcare organization policies.

Evaluate and Ensure

1. Evaluate the specimens and ask the surgeon how the specimen is to be handled (fixed or not fixed with a preservative).
2. Evaluate special handling of the following:
    - Forensic evidence
        - Avoid dropping bullets into metal basins. Only handle using rubber-tipped forceps.
        - Avoid rinsing the evidence.
        - Capture photographic evidence as directed by the surgeon.
        - Change gloves after touching the specimen.
        - Collect evidence as soon as possible.
        - Document the time of collection and where the evidence was taken from the patient's body.
        - Prevent the disposal of potential evidence.
        - Use measuring devices as indicated by the surgeon.
        - Use a standardized forensic evidence collection kit.
3. Highly infectious material
    - Reduce the risk of exposure by alerting all healthcare professionals who might come in contact with the material (i.e., laboratory personnel, other surgical team members).
    - Remove gloves and sanitize hands following the transfer of the specimen.
    - Use standard precautions and PPE when handling all material.
4. Mohs procedure specimens
    - Ensure that high-quality photographs are taken using a ruler, anatomic landmarks, and varied views under the guidance of the surgeon.
5. Placental tissue
    - Patients may request to retrieve placental tissue associated with live birth and related to cultural practices.
    - Handle the specimen according to facility policy and ensure that it is refrigerated until it can be transferred to the pathology laboratory.
6. Prion disease specimens
    - Notify pathology laboratory, sterile processing, and all surgical personnel who will be involved with the case when a patient with prion disease (i.e., CJD) is scheduled.
    - Perform in-person specimen handovers to pathology personnel.
    - Use standard precautions and PPE when handling all materials associated with the case.
7. Radioactive specimens
    - Contain the specimen to prevent cross contamination.
    - Minimize the amount of handling involved.
    - Perform prompt transport of the specimen to the pathology laboratory and in accordance with facility policy.
    - Record the presence of radioactive material on pathology requisition documentation.

 ALERT!

AORN identified ALARA as a mnemonic to be used when handling radioactive specimens. ALARA = **A**s **L**ow **A**s **R**easonably **A**chievable.

8. Umbilical cord blood
  - Follow the facility policy for banked umbilical cord blood.
  - Verify the disposition of umbilical cord blood and whether it is to be banked.
9. Use of formalin
  - Handling of specimens in formalin should follow facility policy and OSHA guidelines. *Formalin is a clear solution of formaldehyde in water.* A 37% solution is used for fixing and preserving biologic specimens for pathologic and histologic examination.
  - Most specimens should be covered in formalin; however, some should not. They are as follows:
    - ○ Calculus
    - ○ Frozen section biopsies
    - ○ Hardware removed from the patient
    - ○ Leg, finger, toe, or arm amputation
    - ○ Lymph node biopsy
    - ○ Muscle or nerve biopsy
  - Logging of the specimen should be completed according to facility policy.
  - Cultures should be handled appropriately.
    - ○ Anaerobic cultures should be placed in the fixative within 10 minutes after the surgeon swabs the affected area.
    - ○ Cotton swabs should not lay on the table for an extended period of time.
    - ○ Cultures should be handled according to facility policy.
  - Specimens (tissue, fluid, bone, hardware) should be immediately passed off the field and placed in a labeled specimen container.
    - ○ Fresh specimens should be delivered to the lab as soon as possible.
    - ○ Frozen section biopsies should be sent to the laboratory upon removal and the time documented on the perioperative record.
    - ○ The process for limb disposal should be followed according to facility policy.

 POP QUIZ 4.5

A 78-year-old male patient has been transferred to the OR for a right colectomy and lymph node excision. Near the end of the procedure, the scrub person notifies the circulating nurse that the specimens are ready for the handoff. The surgeon uses a suture to identify specific margins associated with the tumor removed in the colon. The scrub nurse hands off the colon specimen and the excised tumor in one bowl. The circulating nurse notices the markings on the tumor. What should the nurse do?

RESOURCES

21 CFR 1271. (2017). *Human cells, tissues, and cellular and tissue-based products.* Government Publishing Office.
Apple, B., & Letvak, S. (2021). Ergonomic challenges in the perioperative setting. *AORN Journal, 113*(4), 339–348. http://doi.org/10.1002/aorn.13345
Association for periOperative Registered Nurses. (2013a). *Recommended practices for maintaining a sterile field, Perioperative standards and recommended practices.* Author.
Association for periOperative Registered Nurses. (2013b). *Recommended practices for prevention of retained surgical items, Perioperative standards and recommended practices.* Author.
Association for periOperative Registered Nurses. (2015). *Position statement: Preventing wrong-patient, wrong-site, wrong-procedure events [Toolkit].* https://www.aorn.org/guidelines/clinical-resources/tool-kits/correct-site-surgery-tool-kit
Association for periOperative Registered Nurses. (2019). *Guideline essentials: Key takeaways.* https://www.aorn.org/essentials/team-communication
Association for periOperative Registered Nurses. (2020). *Guideline for surgical attire, Guidelines for perioperative practice.* Author.
Association for periOperative Registered Nurses. (2021a). *AORN correct site surgery tool kit.* https://www.aorn.org/guidelines/clinical-resources/tool-kits/correct-site-surgery-tool-kit

Association for periOperative Registered Nurses. (2021b). *Guideline for a safe environment of care, Guidelines for perioperative practice.* Author.

Association for periOperative Registered Nurses. (2021c). *Guideline for autologous tissue management, Guidelines for perioperative practice.* Author.

Association for periOperative Registered Nurses. (2021d). *Specimen management, Guidelines for perioperative practice.* Author.

Hauk, L. (2018). Guideline for safe patient handling and movement. *AORN Journal, 107,* P10–P12. https://doi.org/10.1002/aorn.12287

Hughes, N. L., Nelson, A., Matz, M. A., & Lloyd, J. (2011). Safe patient handling and movement series. AORN ergonomic tool 4: Solutions for prolonged standing in perioperative settings. *AORN Journal, 93*(6), 767–774. https://doi.org/10.1016/j.aorn.2010.08.029

The Joint Commission. (2021a). *Summary data of sentinel events reviewed by The Joint Commission.* https://www.jointcommission.org/-/media/tjc/documents/resources/patient-safety-topics/sentinel-event/summary-se-report-2020.pdf

The Joint Commission. (2021b). *The universal protocol.* https://www.jointcommission.org/standards/universal-protocol/

Potter, P.A., & Perry, A.G. (2013). Care of the surgical patient. In P.A. Potter & A.G. Perry (Eds.), *Fundamentals in nursing* (8th ed., pp. 1254–1294). Elsevier/Mosby.

Rothrock, J. C. (2018). *Alexander's care of the patient in surgery* (16th ed.). Elsevier - Health Sciences Division.

Quality and Safety Education for Nurses. (2012). *Quality and safety competencies.* http://www.qsen.org/competencies.php

Spera, P., Lloyd, J. D., Hernandez, E., Hughes, N., Peterson, C., Nelson, A., & Spratt, D. G. (2011). Safe patient handling and movement series. AORN ergonomic tool 5: Tissue retraction in the perioperative setting. *AORN Journal, 94*(1), 54–58. https://doi.org/10.1016/j.aorn.2010.08.031

Waters, T., Short, M., Llyod, J., Baptiste, A., Butler, L., Petersen, C., & Nelson, A. (2011). Safe patient handling and movement series. AORN ergonomic tool 2: Positioning and repositioning the supine patient on the OR bed. *AORN Journal, 93*(4), 445–449. https://doi.org/10.1016/j.aorn.2010.08.027

Waters, T., Spera, P., Peterson, C., Nelson, A., Hernandez, E., & Applegarth, S. (2011a). Safe patient handling and movement series. AORN ergonomic tool 3: Lifting and holding the patient's legs, arms, and head while prepping. *AORN Journal, 93*(5), 589–592. https://doi.org/10.1016/j.aorn.2010.08.028

Waters, T., Spera, P., Peterson, C., Nelson, A., Hernandez, E., & Applegarth, S. (2011b). Safe patient handling and movement series. AORN ergonomic tool 7: Pushing, pulling, and moving equipment on wheels. *AORN Journal, 94*(3), 254–260. https://doi.org/10.1016/j.aorn.2010.09.035

INTRAOPERATIVE PERSONNEL AND SERVICES

- There are many people involved in a surgical case. The role of the perioperative nurse is associated with the management of the case's personnel and services.
- This chapter focuses on the function of the interdisciplinary team and the role that the nurse plays in managing personnel and visitors.
- This chapter also includes a discussion of conflict management and the promotion of effective team collaboration and communication.
- Throughout each phase of the perioperative experience, the nurse will perform duties using the ACE process:
  - Assess
  - Confirm
  - Evaluate and Ensure

FUNCTION OF THE INTERDISCIPLINARY TEAM

The interdisciplinary team functions to promote patient care, safety in the environment, and positive patient outcomes. An interdisciplinary surgical team may consist of, but is not limited to, the following personnel:

- Anesthesia personnel
  - Anesthesiologist
    - Function: Provide anesthesia to the patient and support the patient, in conjunction with the CRNA or alone, throughout the procedure through pharmacologic and physiologic intervention.
  - CRNA
    - Function: Provide anesthesia to the patient and support the patient throughout the procedure through pharmacologic and physiologic intervention. In some states, CRNAs are supervised by a physician.
- Biomedical technicians
  - Function: Provide support through maintenance of equipment and routine surveillance and testing of all mechanical equipment.
- Blood salvage technician
  - Function: Operate the cell salvage equipment, maintain the equipment in conjunction with biomedical services, and report blood collection and critical issues to the surgeon and anesthesia personnel.
- Endoscopy technicians
  - Function: Provide support to the physician of record (gastroenterologist) or surgeon during the case and maintain endoscopic equipment and camera sources.
- Materials management personnel
  - Function: Stock sterile materials, place orders for materials used in surgery to achieve preset par levels, and communicate to the OR manager and appropriate team members.

(continued)

FUNCTION OF THE INTERDISCIPLINARY TEAM (continued)

- Sterile core technician or nurse
  - Function: Maintain sterile stock orders, assemble case carts with supplies for scheduled cases, order special equipment as needed, and work with materials management personnel when there are delays in receiving materials needed for surgical cases per facility policy and procedure.
- Surgical assistants
  - Role: Medical assistant, RNFA, PA, APRN, NP, or surgical resident
  - Function: Support the surgeon during the procedure and may perform surgical incision closure, depending upon the scope of practice for the state where the individual is practicing.
- Non-OR personnel
  - Role: HCIR, student observers, and medical residents
  - Function: No formal role or function; HCIRs may offer guidance and instruction on the use of medical equipment and instrumentation.
  - Restrictions: Not permitted to touch any equipment, patient, or open any materials used in a procedure.
- Nurses
  - Preoperative or intraoperative nurse (facility dependent)
    - Function: Perform a presurgical check of all paperwork and a patient assessment.
  - Circulating nurse
    - Function: Maintain the activities in the surgical suite, ensure safety, perform nonsterile functions (open sterile products, materials, and instrumentation), coordinate documents, communicate throughout the procedure, and connect all equipment that exists outside the sterile field.
  - Scrub nurse
    - Function: Maintain the sterile field; receive sterile products, materials, and instruments; and directly assist the surgeon through the passing of instruments and sterile product.
    - Scrub personnel may not always be an RN.
  - RNFA
    - Function: Assist the surgeon with preoperative and postoperative patient management and directly assist with intraoperative surgical management of the patient, including handling of instruments, cutting, closing, and other functions as assigned by the surgeon.
- Nursing assistive personnel
  - Anesthesia technicians
    - Function: Provide support for the anesthesia personnel as assigned under the guidance and supervision of the anesthesiologist and nurse anesthetist.
  - Nursing assistive and OR technicians
    - Assistive personnel roles and official titles are facility dependent.
    - Duties delegated to assistive personnel assigned under guidance and supervision of an RN and in accordance with state nurse practice acts.
  - Other emerging roles: Surgical liaison, robotics coordinator, and nurse informaticist.
    - Function: Support the surgical team in providing patient care through their areas of specialization.
- Perfusionist
  - Function: Operate extracorporeal circulation equipment (heart-lung machine) during open-heart surgery or any other procedure where artificial cardiac support is needed.
- Sterile processing technicians (also known as central service technicians)
  - Function: Prevent infection through sterilization, cleaning, processing, assembling, storing, and distributing the supplies to be used in surgery.
- Surgeon
  - Function: Evaluate, diagnose, and treat conditions through surgical intervention.
- Surgical technologists (also known as OR technicians)
  - Function: Assist the surgeon by providing instrumentation, sharps, equipment, and other sterile materials.

Assess

1. Assess the scope and practice function of each licensed and nonlicensed member of the surgical team.

2. Assess the communication and collaboration efforts of the surgical team.

Confirm

1. Confirm that the appropriate staffing is present in the surgical suite before transfer of the patient from preoperative holding, emergency department, or critical care unit.

2. Confirm that the staffing for a surgical procedure is case dependent and may vary. Standard staffing for a surgical case is as follows:
  - Anesthesia provider (during induction)
  - Circulating nurse
  - RNFA
  - Scrub technician or nurse
  - Surgeon

3. Confirm that the appropriate staffing is present for handoff before and after the surgical case. Staffing is as follows, according to the surgical phase:
  - Preoperative: At least one RN
  - Intraoperative: One RN (circulating nurse) and one scrub person (who may be an RN or surgical technologist)
  - Postoperative Phase I: Two licensed nurses, possibly an RN and RN anesthetist
  - Postoperative Phase II: Two personnel, one should be an RN
  - Phase III and Discharge: One RN (note that this phase occurs beyond the OR and is associated with inpatient status)

4. Confirm that no visitors or HCIRs are in the surgical suite until the patient is prepped and draped for the procedure unless otherwise needed by the surgical team or surgeon.

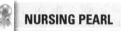 **ALERT!**

Limit all traffic within the surgical suite to only those who need to be present for the case. Limiting activity reduces the risk of SSI.

Evaluate and Ensure

The perioperative RN will evaluate and ensure as follows:

NURSING PEARL

To ensure a high level of quality and standard of care, the circulator must always be an RN and work within the standard of practice identified by the state board of nursing, in accordance with facility policy and AORN recommendations for practice.

1. Evaluate the credentials of the surgical team and the HCIR to determine whether each meets the credentialing requirements for the case and facility, respectively.

2. Ensure the following sterile field management activities are maintained in collaboration with all surgical team members:
  - Check all items on the sterile field are considered sterile.
  - Properly place all items on the sterile field so that they will be subject to minimal movement during the procedure.
  - Properly test all equipment before use to prevent unnecessary delays in the case.
  - Prevent manipulation of sterile items by placing items in a specific place during setup.
  - Plan ahead the position of function for C-arm, laser, or microscope.
  - Place items as close to the area where they will be used as possible.
  - Secure cords and cables to prevent slippage in the sterile field.
  - Work to prevent clutter on and off the sterile field.

3. Promote a culture of safety by acting as follows:
  - Encourage honesty; encourage team members to speak up when errors are present.
  - Engage in conflict resolution processes to improve relationships.

(continued)

Evaluate and Ensure *(continued)*

- Enhance collaboration through effective communication and shared governance.
- Foster a learning culture.
- Maintain and foster adequate leadership and staffing ratios.
- Promote behaviors that are respectful and blameless and that improve teamwork.

4. If applicable, ensure the following related to the HCIR's presence in the case:
- Appropriate surgical attire and an identification badge are worn.
- Individual is not in direct contact with the patient or the patient's medical record.
- Instrumentation and any loaned equipment are approved by the healthcare organization and comply with the manufacturer's terminal sterilization guidelines.
- Participation is based on hospital/organization policy and procedure.
- Patient is made aware of the staff members on the surgical team, including the HCIR.
- Patient's dignity, privacy, safety, and confidentiality are safeguarded at all times.
- Requirement for the individual to be in the room is determined by the nature of the procedure, the surgeon, and the staff (instrument assembly and calibration) and is in compliance with accreditation requirements and local, state, and federal regulations.

POP QUIZ 5.1

The orthopedic surgeon requests that one of the nursing assistive personnel scrubs in to hold retraction on the knee during a right total knee arthroplasty. What should the nurse do?

MANAGEMENT OF PERSONNEL AND SERVICES

The following are the RN's goals for managing personnel and services in the perioperative suite:
- Encourage safety through appropriate staffing. AORN recommends the following parameters for surgical procedure staffing:
  - A minimum of one perioperative RN should be dedicated to performing in the surgical procedure.
  - The perioperative RN supervises, evaluates, and delegates tasks using clinical reasoning skills.
  - The perioperative staffing policy should identify the number of nursing personnel needed by the case based on the complexity of the procedure, team member competencies, patient acuity, monitoring needs, evidence of trauma, and the use of other complex technologies.
  - The staffing plan should include provisions for unplanned, urgent, or emergent procedures and not require the RN to work for more than 12 consecutive hr in a 24-hr period.
  - Staffing level should be set to limit traffic within the perioperative suite.
- Limit the number of personnel in the perioperative suite to only those directly associated with the surgical case.
- Maintain the surgical schedule. Turnover time is the time from the patient leaving the surgical suite to the time of the next patient's arrival.
  - The first case of the day is defined as the time when the first patient scheduled for the OR suite enters the room.
  - Achieving minimal turnover time reduces costs and delays.
  - Surgeon time is associated with the time that the surgeon of record is in the room.
  - Total case time extends from the time set-up in the room for the case to begin until cleanup is complete.
- Maintain patient confidentiality.
- Promote effective communication among the members of the interdisciplinary team.
- Reduce the risk of infection to the patient.
- Reduce the risk of safety issues associated with the movement of patients and equipment.
- Reduce costs associated with providing services to the patient through the following steps:
  - Open only those necessary sterile supplies, devices, medications, and implants confirmed with the surgeon.

- Regularly review physician preference lists, procedural packs, instrument sets, and other equipment sets to remove items that are not used.
- Standardize waste management processes.

UNFOLDING SCENARIO 5A

The general surgeon arranges with the OR manager to have a medical resident observe a laparoscopic cholecystectomy. The circulator asks the visitor the following questions:
- Have you observed in the OR before?
  - The resident states that this is their first time observing.
- Have you eaten today?
  - The resident states that they just had lunch.
- Do you have to go to the restroom?
  - The resident states that they visited the restroom after lunch.

The circulating nurse escorts the resident to a position in the OR suite where they can see the monitors clearly and be out of the traffic perimeter set by the team. The time-out is called by the circulating nurse, at which point the resident moves closer to the sterile field.

Question
What is the circulating nurse's next step?

UNFOLDING SCENARIO 5B

The general surgeon makes the initial incision and inserts the trocars. Insufflation of the abdomen begins. The circulator scans the suite and notices that the resident is swaying back and forth.

Question
What is the circulating nurse's next step?

Assess

1. Assess room preparation.
   - Case cart
     - Assign or delegate an appropriate staff member to check the case carts against the surgeon's preference list and the procedures scheduled for the surgical suite.
     - Develop a consistent process related to the way case supplies (materials, instruments, and equipment for the case) are pulled.
     - Evaluate the surgeon's preference list for completeness and identify the needs for upcoming cases.
   - Equipment
     - Assign or delegate an appropriate staff member to gather equipment.
     - Minimize the need to move equipment from room to room.
     - Use a standardized list of equipment for the surgical suite where feasible.
2. Assess personnel staffing assigned to the case.
   - Personnel
     - Assign or delegate float staff to assist with the turnover of the room, opening cases, providing breaks, and working to support the case from the sterile core.
     - Utilize assistive personnel to aid in the movement of equipment.

Confirm

1. Confirm that the following key measures are observed before, during, and after the case:
   - Consolidate the back table and organize contents for ease of removal at the end of the case (scrub nurse or technician).
   - Keep the OR suite organized (circulating nurse).
     - Keep all cords, pedals, and waste receptacles organized and placed in a manner that prevents trip and fall.
     - Keep all unused sterile equipment, materials, and products in an area of the suite that will preserve the package integrity until they are needed for use.
   - Notify the postanesthesia recovery unit (or the intensive care unit) of the needs of the patient related to a bed and special equipment.
   - Notify the environmental services team at the end of the case to expedite turnover of the suite.
   - Prevent contamination by observing the team to ensure that clean surgical attire and personal protective equipment are worn within the surgical suite during the opening of a case.

Evaluate and Ensure

The perioperative RN will evaluate and ensure the following:
1. Evaluate the chain of command of members within the interdisciplinary team according to the following standards:
   - Level of the scope of practice for each member working within the environment
   - Organizational chart hierarchy
2. Ensure the OR staffing plan includes the following:
   - Provisions for staffing in the event of unplanned, emergent, and urgent procedures
   - RNs who have not been in direct patient care for more than 12 consecutive hr in a 24-hr period or more than 60 hr in a 7-day work week
   - Strategies to minimize extended work hr related to on-call needs
   - Use of patient acuity and nursing workload guidelines for the delivery of safe patient care and the promotion of safety within the work environment
3. Ensure delegation is performed in a manner that takes into consideration the scope of practice for each assistive support member of the interdisciplinary team.
   - Role and scope of practice for delegation to the anesthesia technician and/or technologist:
     - Role: Anesthesia physician of record and nurse anesthetist (if used)
     - Scope of practice
       - Acquire, prepare, and maintain equipment and supplies used for the administration of anesthesia during a procedure.
       - Maintain monitoring devices through cleaning, sterilization, assembly, calibration, testing, troubleshooting, and routine inspection.
   - Role and scope of practice for the perioperative RN (circulator):
     - Perform direct care duties, including the following:
       - Assist with patient care during induction and emergence.
       - Insert catheters.
       - Assess and identify patient.
       - Position the patient.
       - Identify and prepare surgical site.
     - Perform indirect care duties, including the following:
       - Anticipate the needs of the surgical case.
       - Maintain accountability for time-out, documentation, implant handling, specimen handling, patient advocacy, and sterile equipment and products.
       - Control noise, foot traffic, and movement within the environment.
       - Coordinate all elements of patient care.
       - Maintain and monitor temperature and humidity of the environment.
       - Monitor and manage clean air delivery.

- – *Conventional turbulent airflow*: Normal forced air delivered through a standard HVAC system
- – *Unidirectional ultraclean air delivery system (laminar flow)*: HEPA delivered through a steady on-direction stream
- Monitor the surgical environment for breaks in sterility.
- Open sterile supplies and equipment.
- Role and scope of practice for the perioperative RN (scrub nurse or scrub personnel):
  - Perform direct care duties, including the following:
    - Identify and prepare surgical site.
  - Perform indirect care duties, including the following:
    - Anticipate the needs of the surgical case.
    - Maintain accountability for time-out, documentation, implant handling, specimen handling, patient advocacy, and sterile equipment and products.
    - Control noise, foot traffic, and movement within the environment.
    - Coordinate all elements of patient care.
    - Monitor the surgical environment for breaks in sterility.
    - Open sterile supplies and equipment.
    - Safely handle all sharps and sterile equipment.
- Role and scope of practice for the delegation of tasks associated with the nursing assistive personnel (e.g., patient care technician or nurses aid) in the surgical suite:
  - Assist with the movement of equipment and positioning aids needed for the procedure.
  - Perform delegated tasks under the direction of the circulating nurse.
- Role and scope of practice for the HCIR:
  - Adhere to protocols related to limiting of traffic within the OR suite, handling of protected patient information, and adhering to safety precautions as outlined by the facility's policy and procedures.
  - Wear appropriate personal protective equipment in all areas associated with the OR and individual suite.
  - Provide support services, information, and education on medical devices, implants, and products.
  - Provide proof of vendor clearance following the facility's policy.
  - Work under the direction and guidance of the circulating nurse. A circulator may ask the HCIR to retrieve one of the instrument sets that is needed for the case. HCIRs are not permitted to open instrument sets.

4. Ensure that the perioperative efficiency tool kit, created by AORN in 2016, is followed to establish effective patient and equipment flow as listed as follows in the order of occurrence:
- Consent and documentation are complete
- Assessment is performed; patient care and positioning needs are addressed
- Patient arrival to the OR is not delayed and occurs according to the preset OR schedule
- The patient is positioned promptly and in a safe manner
- Assistance is provided to the anesthesia personnel during induction
- Setup of room continues until the time-out process begins

 NURSING PEARL

AORN created the Perioperative Efficiency Tool Kit to educate perioperative nurses on ways to improve preoperative preparation, reduce delays in surgical start times, and improve operational efficiency associated with the workflow from the sterile processing department through the activities in the OR.

 POP QUIZ 5.2

Following the assessment of the patient's chart for the presence of history and physical examination, consents for surgery, anesthesia, blood transfusion, and laboratory results, a patient is transported to the OR for a right total hip arthroplasty. The anesthesia personnel induce the patient, and the surgical site is prepped. The scrub person is gathering sterile drapes to begin draping the patient. The HCIR is in the suite walking around the sterile field. What is the circulating nurse's next step?

(continued)

Evaluate and Ensure *(continued)*

- Assistance is provided to the anesthesia personnel during the patient's emergence from anesthesia
- Equipment and items to be sterilized are promptly transported to their respective areas for cleaning and sterilization
- Cleaning of the perioperative suite occurs swiftly to encourage a prompt turnover
- The patient is safely transported to the recovery unit according to facility policy and by at least two members of the surgical team (i.e., anesthesiologist, certified RN anesthetist, or the circulating nurse)

CONFLICT MANAGEMENT

- The OR is a stressful and isolated department in a hospital setting. Isolation is maintained because the area is kept clean and without clutter in the peripheral areas and sterile within the actual surgical suites. The staff must change into standardized clothes before their entry into this area. This area is prone to the incidence and occurrence of disruptive behaviors and interpersonal conflict.
- The following are the key points of concern related to disruptive behaviors:
  - Occurrence of incident
  - Person(s) perpetrating the incident
  - Nursing perceptions related to impaired clinical decision-making after experiencing disruptive behaviors
  - Patient safety errors related to disruptive behaviors
- Conflict management is an ongoing process in the perioperative environment. The effective management of conflict includes the following steps:
  - Meet face to face with the people involved in the conflict.
  - Avoid a blaming culture and cultivate one that promotes learning.
  - Encourage an environment of collaboration and communication among team members.
  - Improve work environment continuity through reduction of distractions and avoidance of negative behaviors.

Assess

- Assess the type and level of incivility present in the work environment, including the following:
  - Downward violence or disruptive behaviors
    - Abusive behaviors directed at lower-ranked staff from higher-ranked staff (i.e., surgeon to circulating nurse)
    - Throwing of items
    - Verbal abuse
  - Lateral violence
    - Nonverbal expressions
    - Undermining behaviors (i.e., gossip, sabotage, invasion of privacy)
    - Verbal confrontation
- Assess root causes associated with workplace conflict, including the following:
  - Embedded hierarchies
  - Fatigue
  - Ineffective communication
  - Role confusion
  - Stress related to the type of work and challenging procedures
  - Workload

Confirm

Confirm that the following measures are taken:
- Encourage the promotion of respect and collaboration among team members.
- Foster learning within the environment.

 ALERT!

Establishing a blame-free and patient-centered safety culture is a systems-level intervention that improves patient care and outcomes.

- Hold team members accountable for behaviors and actions.
- Observe patient safety goals.
- Promote shared decision-making.
- Reduce barriers to effective communication.

Evaluate and Ensure

- Evaluate the situation and whether workplace violence prevention programs are available at the facility.
- Evaluate and consider the following course of action related to incivility, conflict management, and the promotion of a healthy workplace:
  - Assess one's own actions related to incivility.
  - Engage in ongoing training related to conflict management and healthy workplace promotion.
  - Remain aware of environmental controls and policies that exist to prevent and reduce conflict and violent incidents.
  - Report issues using a standardized reporting protocol and system and in accordance with facility policy and procedure.
  - Take action to initiate change and deescalate the situation if possible.
  - Understand the importance of becoming aware of threatening situations and potential for violence.
- Ensure active participation in conflict reduction in the workplace by:
  - Adhering to the following provisions in the American Nurses Association Code of Ethics:
    - Provision 1: Practicing with compassion and respect for others
    - Provision 3: Promoting and advocating for the patient
    - Provision 5: Preserving the wholeness of character
    - Provision 6: Establishing an ethical environment of care
  - Engaging in continuous improvement activities that foster team collaboration and communication
  - Participating in postevent meetings
  - Providing support to team members
  - Utilizing counseling resources at the facility

POP QUIZ 5.3

The orthopedic surgeon asks the HCIR to get the new bone cement that they had talked about earlier in the day. The circulating nurse alerts the surgeon that the cement has not gone through the appropriate approvals for use according to facility policy. A conflict arises between the surgeon and the nurse, with the surgeon insisting on using the cement. What should the circulating nurse do?

VISITORS

The perioperative nurse is charged with supervising all visitors in the surgical suite. The presence of visitors in the surgical suite should be limited.

Assess

Assess the following associated with visitors to the surgical suite:
- Approval for visitation granted by leadership
- Need for access to other personnel (e.g., HCIR and the scrub personnel)
- Position in the suite
- Presence of appropriate scrub attire, personal protective equipment, and a facility-approved identification badge
- Prior experience of presence in the OR
- Reason for presence in the suite

ALERT!

In some facilities, the visitor may need to have an approval signed by the patient. The perioperative nurse should adhere to the facility policy on visitors in the surgical suite.

Confirm

- Confirm that the patient has been made aware that there will be visitors in the surgical suite and the reason for their presence.
- Confirm that all visitors understand the following:
  - All patient information is to be kept confidential.
  - There should be no physical movement during the time-out process.
- Confirm that visitors have eaten before being in the room and that they know what to do if they feel faint.

Evaluate and Ensure

- Evaluate the suite routinely to ensure that movement within the area is limited, noise is reduced, and traffic is kept to a minimum.
- Ensure the following safety and traffic control interventions are implemented:
  - Create signage indicating specific safety guidelines to be observed (e.g., laser in use, isolation case, latex allergy).
  - Develop language to be used for nonessential visitors when asking them to leave the suite.
  - Educate visitors on the appropriate exit and entry areas (i.e., limit access to the sterile core).
  - Protect the sterile field from contamination and compromise by setting a clear perimeter for visitors to walk around.

> **NURSING PEARL**
>
> The nurse is the first line of defense for patients. Remaining vigilant in one's advocacy for patients and their safety is a top priority.

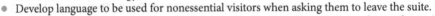

RESOURCES

American Nurses Association. (2015). *American Nurses Association position statement on incivility, bullying, and workplace violence.* https://www.nursingworld.org/~49d6e3/globalassets/practiceandpolicy/nursing-excellence/incivility-bullying-and-workplace-violence--ana-position-statement.pdf

Association for periOperative Registered Nurses. (2013). Recommended practices for maintaining a sterile field. In *Perioperative standards and recommended practices.* Author.

Association for periOperative Registered Nurses. (2016). *AORN perioperative efficiency tool kit* [Toolkit]. https://www.aorn.org/-/media/aorn/guidelines/tool-kits/perioperative-efficiency/aorn-perioperative-efficiency-tool-kit-webinar.pdf?la=en

Association for periOperative Registered Nurses. (2018). Guideline for a safe environment of care. In *Guidelines for perioperative practice.* Author.

Association for periOperative Registered Nurses. (2019a). AORN position statement perioperative registered nurse circulator dedicated to every patient undergoing an operative or other invasive procedure. In *Guidelines for perioperative practice.* Author.

Association for periOperative Registered Nurses. (2019b). *Guideline essentials: Key takeaways.* https://www.aorn.org/essentials/team-communication

Association for periOperative Registered Nurses. (2020a). AORN position statement on allied health care providers and support personnel in the perioperative practice setting. In *Guidelines for perioperative practice.* Author.

Association for periOperative Registered Nurses. (2020b). AORN position statement on perioperative safe staffing and on-call practices. In *Guidelines for perioperative practice.* Author.

Association for periOperative Registered Nurses. (2020c). AORN position statement on the role of the health care industry representative in perioperative settings. In *Guidelines for perioperative practice.* Author.

Association for periOperative Registered Nurses. (2021). *Re-entry guidance for health care facilities and medical device representatives.* https://www.aorn.org/guidelines/aorn-support/re-entry-guidance-for-health-care-facilities

Link, T. (2018). A postprocedure wrap-up tool for improving OR communication and performance. *AORN Journal, 108*(2). https://doi.org/10.1002/aorn.12007

Mews, P. A., & Wafer, P. (2020). *Perioperative efficiency: Patient safety, workflow, and quality. AORN: Safe surgery together toolkit.* Association for periOperative Registered Nurses.

Norton, B., & Mordas, D. (2018). A postprocedure wrap-up tool for improving OR communication and performance. *AORN Journal, 107*(1), 108–115. https://doi.org/10.1002/aorn.12300

COMMUNICATION AND DOCUMENTATION

- Creating a patient safety culture requires effective team collaboration and communication. Written communication through documentation also aids in safeguarding the patient while promoting effective and efficient care. This chapter emphasizes the following aspects of perioperative nursing:
  - Effective hand-off protocols and documentation to facilitate communication, workflow, and patient safety
  - Employment of methods to enhance quality
  - Promotion of respect among team members
  - The role of education in developing a patient safety culture
- Throughout each phase of the perioperative experience, the nurse will perform duties using the ACE process:
  - Assess
  - Confirm
  - Evaluate and Ensure

COMMUNICATION AMONG CAREGIVERS

- Communication among caregivers in the perioperative setting is vital to maintaining the safety of patients and staff and reducing barriers to team collaboration.
- Communication issues have been identified as a root cause for sentinel events that occur during surgery and range from wrong-patient and wrong-site events to wrong-procedure events that cause harm to the patient.

Assess

Assess the following potential communication barriers:
- High noise levels within the perioperative suite
- Impediments to exchange of dialogue due to equipment or layout of the surgical suite
- Irrelevant conversation among the team members
- Nonessential activity or movement (during time-out, critical conversations between team members, induction, emergence, counting, and specimen handling)
- Patient's language barriers or nonverbal status

Confirm

- Confirm that the members of the perioperative team maintain a patient safety culture through the following strategies:
  - Accountability for behaviors in the OR suite
  - Adequacy of staffing
  - Adherence to the pillars of safety (trust, report, and improve)

(continued)

Confirm (continued)

- Appreciation of members' contributions to the team
- Attentiveness and cessation of all activity during the time-out
- Commitment to voicing safety concerns
- Encouragement of honesty
- Promotion of a learning culture
- Confirm that the following information is communicated to the interdisciplinary healthcare team members involved in the patient's care:
  - Communication needs of the patient
  - Implants or implanted device location
  - Medications used during surgery
  - Report of allergies
  - Status of the patient's medical condition during and at the end of surgery (e.g., breaks in sterility, fluid losses, blood loss, and urine output)

ALERT!

Speaking up can save lives. Encourage a culture of safety for everyone.

Evaluate and Ensure

- Evaluate potential and actual systems failures that undermine a culture of safety associated with the surgical team, including the following:
  - Deviation from standards of practice or errors in practice
  - Interpersonal conflicts
  - Lapses in judgment
  - Mistakes in practice

NURSING PEARL

Communication is one of the most vital components of a nurse's toolbox. Use effective communication to promote team collaboration, reduce incivility in the work environment, and improve patient outcomes.

- Ensure effective communication and collaboration by doing the following:
  - Address behaviors that could lead to harm of the patient or create barriers in the work environment.
  - Ensure that a standardized briefing process, known as the *universal protocol*, is used during each of the operative phases.
  - Ensure adequate staff is available to move the patient at the end of the procedure.
  - Monitor and cross-check processes and procedures used in practice.
  - Read back and verify when
    - needing clarity,
    - receiving critical information on a patient,
    - dispensing medications or fluids to the field by the circulator to the scrub nurse, and
    - receiving medication or other orders from the surgeon or anesthesiologist.
  - Use clear, specific, and concise descriptions of tasks to be delegated or needs of the case.
  - Use the chain of command and standardized process when reporting issues.
  - Use a standardized process, tools, and chain of command when
    - reporting patient information related to adverse event issues,
    - needing a team debriefing at the end of a procedure or after an adverse event,
    - transferring care to the receiving unit (e.g., PACU, ICU)
    - transferring care to relief staff, and
    - voicing concerns as they arise.

POP QUIZ 6.1

A 50-year-old male is transported to the OR from the preoperative holding area to undergo an arteriovascular graft for dialysis. The graft product is opened without verifying the expiration. The circulating nurse notices that the product is expired just prior to the surgeon inserting the graft. The circulating nurse alerts the surgeon that the product is expired. What could have prevented this error?

UNFOLDING SCENARIO 6A

A 58-year-old metal worker enters the OR for the removal of a mass in their left upper scapular area under general anesthesia. The patient's history and physical examination review reveals that there is a 40-year history of smoking, COPD, and hypertension. The patient's height is documented as 70 in, and the weight is 265 lb.

The patient is not yet sedated and is able to move onto the OR bed and lie in the supine position. The anesthesia provider confers with the surgeon on whether the patient should be positioned in the right lateral position to maintain the compromised airway. The surgeon responds, "Sure," and leaves it to the scrub person. The anesthesia provider begins induction with assistance from the circulating nurse.

The circulating nurse then gathers the pillows and axillary roll and stands by the patient's side while loosening the safety strap. The anesthesia provider helps the circulating nurse shift the patient to lie on their right side with the knees bent until comfortable and with the right arm extended on an arm board. The nurse places the axillary roll under the right shoulder area and places a pillow between the legs and under the left elbow, which is resting on a Mayo stand. The safety strap is placed over the patient's thighs and attached to the OR table. The circulator confirms with the anesthesia provider that the patient is in a good position.

The circulating nurse proceeds with the prep; there is a little pooling of the iodine-based solution, but because the procedure is so short, the circulator leaves it. After draping is finished, the circulating nurse helps the scrub person move the Mayo stand for additional sterile draping by the scrub person. The scrub person lays the patient's arm on the left side of the body to rest while the Mayo stand is draped, and the back table is repositioned by the scrub person to the left of the surgeon and the incision site. The left arm is then positioned on the sterile-draped Mayo stand.

The circulator calls for the time-out and reads the checklist. All items on the checklist are approved by the team except for allergies. The anesthesia personnel reminds the team that the patient has an allergy to iodine. The case is short, and the surgeon cleans the area around the left upper scapula with sterile saline.

The circulating nurse begins documentation on the electronic health record. Suddenly, the patient's legs slip from the table, the surgeon yells, and contents from the Mayo stand fall. The anesthesia provider removes the drapes to hold the patient and prevent them from slipping down the table. One side of the safety strap had not been securely fastened. The anesthesia provider also notices a rash present on the area of the prepped skin.

Question 1

What errors in communication occurred?

Question 2

How could the injury to the patient have been prevented?

DOCUMENTATION IN THE PATIENT RECORD

The legal health record consists of the documentation of all services, products used for service, medications, plans of care (assessment, diagnosis, planning, implementation, and evaluation), and notes on end-of-life support decisions and advanced directives related to patient care.

Assess

- Assess the patient care record for the following:
  - Complete and accurate informed consent for surgery and anesthesia administration, including the following information:
    - Date (typically must be dated fewer than 30 days prior but depends on facility policy)
    - Name of the healthcare facility, invasive procedure to be performed, and healthcare representative performing the procedure
    - Signatures with date and time of the patient and healthcare provider's signature; if patient unable to sign, signature of legal patient representative

(continued)

Assess *(continued)*

  - ○ Statement of the risks and benefits associated with the proposed procedure and alternatives to the procedure
- Disposition orders for the placenta for live births (facility dependent) and death certificate documentation in the case of fetal demise
- Disposition of limb documentation (for amputation)
- History and physical report (within the last 30 days or according to facility policy)
- Laboratory and radiology reports
- Medication records
- Orders pertaining to the planned procedure
- Other documentation associated with the procedure (e.g., limb disposal consents, blood transfusion consent)
- Assess equipment settings and document initial settings and all changes to settings during the procedure for:
  - Ablation equipment
  - Argon-enhanced coagulation
  - Arthroscopic irrigation equipment
  - Autoclaves
  - Defibrillators
  - Electrosurgical generator
  - Fluid warmers
  - Hysteroscopy pumps
  - Infusion pumps
  - Lasers
  - Light sources
  - Medical gas (e.g., nitrogen)
  - Microscopes
  - Patient warming devices (forced-warm air)
  - Pneumatic tourniquets
  - Sequential compression devices

Confirm

- Confirm that the perioperative record includes documentation of the following according to facility policy and procedure:
  - Notes associated with adverse events or unplanned activities as per facility policy (e.g., retained foreign body, injury to the patient, change from a laparoscopic procedure to an open procedure)
  - Products used during the procedure (including implantable material)
  - Record of explants, implants, and surgical specimens
  - Roles, credentials, and the time present in the perioperative suite for the following:
    - ○ HCIR
    - ○ Law enforcement
    - ○ Observers
    - ○ Perioperative personnel
    - ○ Pathology and radiology staff
    - ○ Support staff
    - ○ Surgeons and assistants
  - Time associated with the following:
    - ○ Administration of antibiotics
    - ○ Transfer of specimens from the surgical field to pathology
    - ○ Removal of specimens from the surgical field and fixative times (if needed)
    - ○ Surgical start and end
    - ○ Time-out process
    - ○ Placement of tourniquet and settings
    - ○ Transport of patient into and out of the surgical suite

UNFOLDING SCENARIO 6B

The case of the 58-year-old metal worker who needed a removal of a mass in their left upper scapular area under general anesthesia has ended, and the patient has been extubated. The circulating nurse and the nurse anesthetist make final adjustments to the patient's position to transfer to the hospital bed. The circulating nurse reassesses the rash and notes that the area is still red.

Question

The circulating nurse finalizes documentation on the electronic health record. What information should the nurse include on the chart?

Evaluate and Ensure

- Evaluate barriers to communication among healthcare team members.
  - Environmental factors
    - ○ Interruptions in the surgical process
    - ○ Multiple conversations
    - ○ Music
    - ○ Noise
  - Human factors
    - ○ Disruptive behavior
    - ○ Embedded hierarchies
    - ○ Fatigue
    - ○ Focus on a specific patient issue or surgical issue
    - ○ Hunger
    - ○ Stress
- Evaluate the documentation tools used in perioperative practice and the downtime process associated with documentation offline.
- Evaluate documentation to ensure compliance with state guidelines and national accreditation requirements related to the following areas:
  - Blood and tissue tracking
  - Implant tracking
  - Infection control practices (e.g., surgical preparation methods and antibiotic prophylaxis)
  - Injury reduction measures (e.g., positioning aids used)
  - Intraoperative testing
  - Medication administration and reconciliation
  - Pain management interventions
  - Patient education (preoperative phase)
  - Urinary catheter insertion
- Ensure that the patient's health record is safeguarded for privacy using the following procedures:
  - Limit the use of mobile devices in the perioperative suite.
  - Minimize the electronic record on the computer screen to restrict access to the patient record during the procedure.
  - Observe guidelines related to the HIPAA of 1996.
  - Protect the paper health record by covering all patient information.
  - Refrain from sharing facility-assigned log-in information with other staff and visitors to the OR unit or individual suite.

NURSING PEARL

An old adage states that, "If you did not document it, you did not do it." Remember to document all activities and actions that occur before and during the procedure and upon transfer to the PACU.

ALERT!

Tissue Tracking

TJC recommends that all staff members coming into contact with any type of tissue, bones, or vessels be tracked and that this tracking be documented according to FDA and AATB requirements.

(continued)

Evaluate and Ensure *(continued)*

- Retain all patient care-related information in its original and legally reproducible format according to facility policy.
- Use the facility-approved platform to access the patient's health record.

- Ensure all pertinent information is documented in the electronic health record or paper chart.
- Ensure that the facility policy related to documentation is followed.
- Ensure communication processes are followed to support continuity of patient care, such as by using one of the following procedures:
  - *IPASS the BATON:* This type of hand-off procedure requires the following information be shared when transferring care to another healthcare provider:
    - *Introduction* of the staff to the patient
    - *Patient name,* identifiers, age, sex, and location of the surgery
    - *Assessment* of vital signs, focused assessment related to surgery
    - *Situation* or circumstances that led to the patient having surgery
    - *Safety* concerns associated with critical lab results, allergies, and positioning
    the
    - *Background information* associated with comorbidities, medications, family, and social history
    - *Actions* that will need to be taken to ensure positive patient outcome
    - *Timing* of actions and the urgency level associated with the surgery
    - *Ownership* of the roles and responsibilities for each aspect of care during the perioperative experience
    - *Next or anticipated changes* and the plan for the surgical team to provide care
  - *SBAR:* This widely known hand-off procedure identifies the four aspects of information needed when reporting off to a relief nurse or another level of care. In perioperative nursing, SBAR is used as follows:
    - *Situation:* Summarizes the situation at a given point in time (i.e., count results at the end of the surgery, status of dressing application, documentation requirements)
    - *Background:* Describes issues that may have occurred during the procedure (contamination of an instrument, person, table, etc.)
    - *Assessment:* Describes how well the patient tolerated the procedure and if there are special considerations (drain placement, tourniquet time, etc.)
    - *Recommendation:* Describes other recommendations for patient care issues that still need attention or require follow-up in the surgical suite
  - *Read Back and Verify:* This procedure requires all perioperative personnel to read back and verify (audibly for all team members) orders from the surgeon and/or delegated tasks, including the following:
    - Deviations from the normal standard of care (i.e., trauma cases, emergencies, disasters)
    - Medications dispensed to the sterile field
    - Positioning of the patient
    - Specimen handling, labeling, documentation, and transport (e.g. tissue, blood, fluid.)
    - Verbal orders from the surgeon or anesthesiologist
  - *Standardized Surgical Checklist:* This checklist is used during the preprocedure check-in, patient sign-in to the surgical suite, time-out, and patient sign-out of the surgical suite and transport to the next level of care.
- Ensure that the documentation associated with tissue tracking is complete and the process adheres to facility, state, and federal guidelines (Table 6.1).
- Ensure that the documentation associated with implants is complete and the process adheres to facility, state, and federal guidelines.

- Ensure the following information is obtained related to autologous tissue according to facility policy:
  - Date of recovery
  - Disposition of the tissue and all those who handle it
  - Name of the surgeon
  - Type of procedure
  - Type of storage and temperature
  - Type of tissue and method of preservation

POP QUIZ 6.2

A patient is transported to the OR from the medical-surgical floor to undergo a right total hip arthroplasty. Once the patient is positioned on the surgical table, the nurse notices erythema and swelling of the right heel not reported during hand-off communication upon the patient's transfer to the OR. What should the nurse do first?

Table 6.1 Tissue Tracking Recommendations and Guidelines

Tissue Type	Storage	Special Considerations

Cranial bone flaps	Frozen, cryopreserved, or in a subcutaneous pocket for replantation	• Facility guidelines should include the method for preparing the bone flap:
		  ◦ Removal of blood and excess tissue
		  ◦ Use of a low-linting sterile material to dry the bone
		  ◦ Use of the sterile technique to prepare the bone for packaging

Femoral head	Can be stored in the iliac pocket	• The storage and preservation of the femoral head in the iliac pocket is associated with total hip arthroplasty revision procedures.
Parathyroid tissue	Cryopreserved or auto-transplanted	• Call ahead to pathology when the tissue is in transit. • Place the specimen in a sterile specimen cup and on sterile ice. • Transport specimen to the pathology lab as soon as possible.
Skin	Preserved or auto-transplanted (i.e., split-thickness graft)	• Preserve the skin through refrigeration according to facility policy and guidelines. • Place the graft on a sheet of tulle gras with the epithelial side down. • Wrap the graft in moistened saline gauze or place it in a sterile container.
Vessels	Preserved or transplanted	• Store in a buffered storage solution or tissue culture medium for no longer than 14 days.

RESOURCES

Agency for Healthcare Research and Quality. (2019, June). *Team STEPPS 2.0.* U.S. Department of Health and Human Services, Agency for Healthcare Research and Quality. https://www.ahrq.gov/teamstepps/instructor/index.html

American Health Information Management Association. (2011, February). Fundamentals of the legal health record and designated record set. *Journal of AHIMA, 82*(2). https://library.ahima.org/doc?oid=104008#.YG9bNuhKiUk

American Nurses Association. (2015). *American Nurses Association position statement on incivility, bullying, and workplace violence.* https://www.nursingworld.org/~49d6e3/globalassets/practiceandpolicy/nursing-excellence/incivility-bullying-and-workplace-violence--ana-position-statement.pdf

Association for periOperative Registered Nurses. (2019). Autologous tissue management. In *Guidelines for perioperative practice.* Author.

Association for periOperative Registered Nurses. (2020a). Information management. In *Guidelines for perioperative practice.* Author.

Association for periOperative Registered Nurses. (2020b). Team communication. In *Guidelines for perioperative practice.* Author.

Link, T. (2018a). Guideline implementation: Team communication. *AORN Journal, 108*(2), 165–177. https://doi.org/10.1002/aorn.12300

Link, T. (2018b). A postprocedure wrap-up tool for improving OR communication and performance. *AORN Journal, 108*(2). https://doi.org/10.1002/aorn.12007

Pradetha, A. (2017, October 9). Meeting joint commission tissue tracking requirements. *Mobile Aspects.* https://www.mobileaspects.com/meeting-joint-commission-tissue-tracking-requirements/

INFECTION PREVENTION AND CONTROL OF ENVIRONMENT, INSTRUMENTATION, AND SUPPLIES

OVERVIEW

- Regulatory and accrediting organizations have stringent requirements around infection prevention, and facilities have mechanisms to prevent infection, but HAIs remain high.
- According to TJC, the incidence of SSIs, one type of HAI, is staggering, with approximately 500,000 cases reported annually.
- Throughout each phase of the perioperative experience, the nurse will perform duties using the ACE process:
  - Assess
  - Confirm
  - Evaluate and Ensure

REGULATORY STANDARDS FOR INFECTION PREVENTION

- The *Guideline for Prevention of Surgical Site Infection* was first published in 1999 by a team of medical doctors and infection control practitioners.
- Healthcare professionals followed these guidelines inconsistently. In response, a national quality improvement standardization project led to the development of the SCIP, a collaboration of the CMS and the CDC. Several SCIP elements focus on preventing SSIs.
- TJC expanded upon these guidelines to develop NPSGs. Specifically, NPSG.07.05.01, *Implement Evidence-Based Practices for Preventing Surgical Site Infections*, specifies standards of practice to prevent SSIs in OR suites, ambulatory care centers, and office-based surgery centers.
- The American College of Surgeons National Surgery Quality Improvement Program provides guidance and analyses on quality improvement processes for participating hospitals.

Assess

- Assess compliance with federal, state, and local regulatory bodies related to infection prevention associated with sharps handling, single-use and reusable products, skin preparation, surgical antibiotic prophylaxis, surgical gloves, urinary catheter use, thermoregulation, and surgical smoke evacuation.
- Assess facility policy and procedures associated with the prevention of SSI.

Confirm

- Confirm that all members of the surgical team are compliant with and adhere to TJC guidelines outlined in the annually updated NPSGs.

(continued)

Confirm *(continued)*

- Confirm that OSHA, CDC, and Joint Commission regulatory standards and AORN professional guidelines associated with infection prevention practices for each of the following are maintained:
  - Blood glucose levels as follows:
    - Cardiac patient: Less than 180 mg/dL
    - Preoperative phase: Less than 200 mg/dL
    - Perioperative phase: Between 110 and 150 mg/dL
  - Nasal decolonization for patients undergoing cardiothoracic, spine, and orthopedic procedures or as indicated by the facility policy
  - Normothermia throughout the surgical procedure with a core temperature above 95 °F (35 °C)
  - Sharps handling and injury prevention
    - Avoid recapping of needles.
    - Confine and contain all sharps in specifically allocated areas of the sterile field or sharps containers off the field.
    - Use an instrument to remove the blade from the blade holder.
    - Use a neutral zone (e.g., basin, instrument mat, magnetic pad, designated area on the Mayo stand) for passing sharps during a surgical case.
    - Use a no-touch technique and avoid sharp edges when handling ampules, needles, K-wires, and blades.
  - Skin preparation before the surgical procedure according to facility policy:
    - Remove hair only if it will interfere with the surgical procedure, and do so only by clipping around the surgical site.
    - Confirm that the patient has followed preoperative bathing protocols.
  - Single-use barrier products
    - Inspect upon donning and before contact with any sterile supplies on the sterile field.
    - Confirm that surgical gowns and drape products provide a barrier to protect the patient and staff from blood-borne pathogens.
    - Confirm that single-use barrier products are resistant to tears and punctures and reduce exposure to other body fluids.
  - Surgical antibiotic prophylaxis
    - Administer according to evidence-based practice guidelines (typically 30 to 60 minutes before surgical incision is made).
  - Surgical gloves
    - Inspect gloves upon donning and before contact with any sterile supplies on the surgical field.
    - Breaches in the glove barrier increase the risk for transmission of blood-borne pathogens and the risk of SSI from contact with nonsterile skin during surgical procedures.
    - Double-gloving reduces the risk of SSI, percutaneous injuries, glove perforation to the inner-most glove, and blood-borne contamination.
  - Surgical smoke toxicity
    - Use appropriate surgical masks and smoke evacuation practices to prevent toxicity from the following particles:
      - Allergens
      - Bio-aerosols
      - Blood
      - Carcinogens
      - Dead and live cellular material
      - Dust
      - Infectious bacteria
      - Neurotoxins
      - Toxic gases and vapors
      - Viruses

 ALERT!

In 2021, multiple states (Illinois, Oregon, Kentucky, Rhode Island, Colorado) passed legislation mandating the use of surgical smoke evacuation.

Evaluate and Ensure

- Evaluate the perioperative environment for any potential sources of infection.
- Ensure adherence to AORN guidelines for transmission-based precautions as follows:
  - Reduce the transmission of bioburden and microbial contamination that may enter the surgical site through the patient's skin, surgical personnel, air, and contaminated surfaces or instrumentation.
  - Use standard precautions when providing patient care.
  - Use contact precautions with patients with known infections or those who are colonized with a pathogen.
  - Wear the appropriate PPE during all patient handling and if it is anticipated that there will be exposure to blood-borne pathogens, infectious material, or bodily fluids.

UNFOLDING SCENARIO 7A

The sterile field is prepped and draped for a dual procedure, an open cholecystectomy and exploratory laparotomy. The scrub personnel establish a neutral zone. During the procedure, the surgeon makes the incision to start the procedure and inadvertently pierces the drape with the knife blade.

Question

What is the purpose of a neutral zone? What should the scrub personnel do in this scenario?

SURGICAL SCRUBBING AND HAND HYGIENE

- Colonization is the asymptomatic carrying of organisms on the skin, in the body fluids, or on the tissues, not causing a clinically adverse effect for an individual.
- Decolonization is the use of antimicrobial or antiseptic agents to suppress or eradicate colonization.
- Perioperative personnel must adhere to strict hand hygiene practices when providing patient care and handling sterile supplies and equipment. This section discusses surgical scrubbing techniques and hand hygiene practices to be followed in the perioperative area.
- Surgical scrubbing uses surgical skin antiseptics to minimize resident flora on the skin, reducing the risk of contamination by microorganisms during operative or invasive procedures.

Assess

- Assess the use of appropriate hand antisepsis by all members of the surgical team:
  - Broad spectrum
  - Fast acting
  - FDA approved
  - Persistent in maintaining the reduction of bacterial colonization at 6 hr
- Assess the use of appropriate techniques and solutions, noting that alcohol-based solutions cannot penetrate spores, and mechanical friction during soap and water handwashing is most effective against spore-forming organisms such as the following:
  - *Clostridium difficile*
  - *Bacillus anthracis*
  - Norovirus
- Assess decolonization protocols, including the following:
  - Evaluate allergies and sensitivities to skin antiseptics.
  - Remove all visible soil and debris from the surgical site using an approved skin antiseptic agent.

(continued)

Assess *(continued)*

- Use intranasal administration of mupirocin in combination with an FDA-approved skin antiseptic agent such as CHG for decolonization.
- Hair should be left at the surgical site unless it is clinically contraindicated.
- Instruct patients to bathe or shower with either soap and water or the prescribed skin antisepsis.

Confirm

- Perioperative personnel should confirm that the following hand hygiene goals are met:
  - Maintain healthy skin.
    - Damaged skin may harbor staphylococci and gram-negative bacilli.
  - Maintain healthy nails.
  - Maintain short nails, length not exceeding 2 mm (0.08 in.) to do the following:
    - Decrease the risk of bacterial colonization beneath the nail
    - Prevent perforation of the surgical gloves
    - Prevent patient injury during transfer
  - Use alcohol-based hand scrub.
  - Use facility-approved moisturizers that are compatible with hand hygiene products to prevent degradation of scrub solutions and breakdown of surgical gloves.
  - Use water that is in the temperature range of 70 °F to 80 °F (21 °C–26.7 °C).
  - Wash hands with soap and water for a minimum of 15 seconds.

 ALERT!

Perioperative personnel must do the following:
- Perform a proper surgical hand scrub as the first line of defense in minimizing pathogens' transmission from the hands to the patient.
- Provide a second line of defense by donning sterile gloves to decrease the risk of SSI.

Evaluate and Ensure

- Evaluate the skin integrity of those who are performing a surgical scrub before the procedure:
  - Personnel with visibly cracked or peeling skin should refrain from scrubbing in for the procedure.
  - Personnel with subcutaneous outbreaks or skin abrasions are less likely to perform appropriate hand hygiene.
- Ensure that the surgical hand scrub (alcohol-based or packaged scrub brush) is performed per the manufacturer's IFU and according to AORN standards for hand hygiene:
  - Don a surgical mask
  - Remove all jewelry from the hands and the wrists
  - Open the scrub brush
  - Turn the water on
  - Remove debris from under the fingernails using the disposable nail cleaner
  - Rinse the hands
  - Use the scrub brush to address all four sides of each hand and each finger according to the manufacturer's recommendation for use
  - Hold the hands higher than the elbows during the scrubbing process
  - Avoid splashing water on surgical attire
  - Rinse the hands by running each arm through the stream in an upward fashion
- Ensure that perioperative personnel perform hand hygiene for activities including, but not limited to, the following:
  - Before and after patient contact, including site marking and wound care, or involving blood or bodily fluids
  - Before and after accessing or handling an invasive device, a vascular device, a urinary catheter, or a colostomy bag
  - Before eating and after using the restroom
  - Before performing a clean or sterile task or after removing PPE

- Ensure that perioperative personnel are not
  - wearing artificial nails or polish that may inhibit the ability to properly perform hand hygiene or interfere with the procedure.
    - Chipped nail polish may contaminate the sterile field with nail polish fragments.
    - Gel nail polish may cause potential damage to the natural fingernail and increase the risk for bacterial colonization in damaged areas of the nail and cuticle.
    - The classification of artificial nails is facility specific; however, some examples of artificial nails include, but are not limited to, the following:
      - Acrylic
      - Artificial bonding material
      - Extensions
      - Gel
      - Overlays
      - Tape
      - Tips
      - Wraps
- Ensure that perioperative personnel
  - Are encouraged to double-glove so that the outer glove can act as an additional barrier that can be removed to avoid delay caused by hand hygiene.
  - Remove gloves after completing patient care activities and performing hand hygiene.
  - Weigh the risks and benefits of wearing gloves during life-saving interventions such as ventilation and airway management.

> **ALERT!**
>
> Artificial nails have been implicated in the spread of gram-negative bacteria and yeast.

UNFOLDING SCENARIO 7B

During the procedure, the abdominal cholecystectomy with exploratory laparotomy is taking longer than scheduled, and it is time for the scrub person to have a lunch break. The relief scrub is at the scrub sink getting ready to scrub in. The circulating nurse checks on the relief scrub and notices that only a quick application of the alcohol-based hand antisepsis product has been completed. The circulating nurse is next to be relieved for lunch. The relief nurse comes into the room noting that her hands are dry. She takes lotion out of her pocket brought from home and applies it to her hands.

Question

How should the circulating nurse intervene with the scrub nurse and the relief nurse?

SURGICAL ATTIRE

Surgical attire consists of the facility-approved scrub shirt and pants, the bouffant cap, and shoe covers. At the surgical field, the attire consists of an additional layer of protection including the surgical gown and eye protection. This section reviews specifics associated with AORN's guideline for surgical attire.

Assess

- Assess the following related to head-to-toe surgical attire requirements:
  - Personal clothing must be
    - Nonlinting
    - Covered by approved scrub attire
    - Laundered daily and when contaminated with blood, bodily fluids, or infectious materials
  - Arms may be covered with long-sleeved, hospital-laundered jackets when performing the patient's surgical skin prep.

(continued)

Assess (continued)

- Head must be covered when entering semi-restricted and restricted areas to avoid shedding hair and bacteria that may contaminate a sterile field.
  - ○ Cloth caps must be clean and laundered according to facility policy.
  - ○ The standard bouffant cap placed over the cloth cap may be an additional requirement in some facilities.
  - ○ Only facility-approved head coverings should be used within the semi-restricted and restricted areas.
  - ○ Perioperative team members should always refer to facility policy.
  - ○ Personnel may wear a head covering for the entire day (all other PPE must be removed when leaving the semi-restricted and restricted areas).
- Jewelry should not be worn. If it is approved to be worn, the following is advised by AORN:
  - ○ Scrubbed personnel must not wear jewelry.
  - ○ Theoretical risk of harm exists since jewelry could come off and contaminate a sterile field or enter a surgical wound.
  - ○ Unscrubbed personnel must keep jewelry to a minimum; however, jewelry impedes the completion of effective hand hygiene.
- The face must be covered.
  - ○ Beards
    - ■ Perioperative personnel should cover beards.
  - ○ Masks must
    - ■ Be worn in restricted areas
    - ■ Be changed if wet or soiled
    - ■ Be changed between patients
    - ■ Be discarded when leaving the restricted area
    - ■ Be secured appropriately
    - ■ **Not** be left to hang near the neck or chest
- The feet should be protected with shoes that are clean and have closed heels and front.

Confirm

Confirm that surgical scrub attire is laundered properly.
- Perioperative personnel cannot easily monitor quality and consistency in home laundering and should use the following guidelines:
  - Do not launder surgical scrub attire at home.
  - Do not place contaminated scrubs in a washer; this may deposit bioburden and transmit microorganisms to other clothing.
  - Do not store surgical scrubs in lockers to wear again.
  - Remove surgical attire before leaving the facility.
  - Wear facility-laundered scrubs washed following state recommendations or CDC guidelines.

Evaluate and Ensure

- Evaluate scrub attire for pilling of fabric, tears, lint, or soiling.
- Ensure that the laundering of surgical attire occurs through an approved vendor selected by the facility.

STANDARD AND TRANSMISSION-BASED PRECAUTIONS

- The CDC identifies two tiers of precautions to be considered when preventing infection in the healthcare setting: Standard and transmission-based precautions.
  - Standard precautions, considered the first tier of precautions, are used for all patients, and are used for patients who are infected or colonized with an infectious agent.
  - Transmission-based precautions are the second tier of infection control and are used in addition to standard precautions.
- The goal of using both standard and transmission-based precautions is to prevent infection transmission to healthcare personnel, patients, and visitors in the facility.

Assess

Assess the patient related to the need for the following precautions:
- Standard precautions: Use standard precautions for all patient care. Follow CDC protocol, which includes
  - Donning appropriate PPE
  - Following respiratory hygiene principles
  - Handling and disinfecting patient care equipment and instruments
  - Performing hand hygiene
- Contact precautions: Use contact precautions when a patient is known to have
  - Group A Streptococcus (*Streptococcus pyogenes*), known as "flesh-eating bacteria"
  - MDRO
- Droplet and airborne precautions: Use droplet or airborne precautions for patients with
  - Adenovirus
  - Coronaviruses (SARS-CoV, MERS-CoV, and SARS-CoV-2)
  - Draining TB lesions
  - Ebola virus
  - Group A Streptococcus infections
  - Smallpox
  - Varicella-zoster virus
- Droplet precautions: Use droplet precautions for
  - Adenovirus, rhinovirus
  - Group A Streptococcus (*S. pyogenes*)
  - Influenza
  - Mumps
  - *Neisseria meningitides* (meningitis)
  - Pertussis (whooping cough)

Confirm

Confirm that all perioperative personnel don the appropriate PPE associated with each type of precaution according to the CDC (2016) guidelines:
- Airborne precautions
  - Gloves
  - Particulate respirator (e.g., N95 or powered air purifying respirator)
- Contact precautions
  - Face mask
  - Gloves
  - Gown
- Droplet precautions
  - Face mask
  - Gloves
  - Eye protection (shields, goggles, glasses)

Evaluate and Ensure

- Evaluate the activity within the perioperative suite, both on and off the sterile field, for biohazardous fluid spills and cross-contamination.
- Evaluate patients for the presence of MDRO or other organisms requiring more than standard precautions. Ensure that the hierarchy of controls to prevent the spread of infection is utilized by perioperative personnel, including
  - Adherence to policy and procedure for isolation and reducing the transmission of disease
  - Elimination of the hazard

 ALERT!

Perioperative personnel should consider each patient's blood and bodily fluids as contagious.

Sweat and tears are not considered contagious. (CDC, 2016)

(continued)

Evaluate and Ensure *(continued)*

- Management of environmental controls (i.e., negative pressure for airborne disease)
- Safe work practice (i.e., safe sharps handling, proper body mechanics)
- Wearing appropriate PPE

UNFOLDING SCENARIO 7C

The surgical case is wrapping up, and final counts are complete. The scrub person begins to remove blades from the handle when a blade slips and slices through both of the gloves on one hand. The circulator calls the charge nurse for an emergency relief scrub.

Question

What should the scrub nurse do?

STANDARDS FOR STERILIZATION OF INSTRUMENTATION

AORN has issued guidelines and standards associated the sterilization of instrumentation. This section will covers some of the newest guidelines and key points.

Assess

- Assess all wrapped packaging for tears, rips, moisture, and sterilization indicators.
- Assess all rigid containers for a proper seal and indication that sterilization parameters have been met.

Confirm

- Confirm that the guidelines for sterile processing personnel are met.
- If sterilization parameters have not been met, confirm the following is completed:
  - Assess whether the failure puts the patient at risk
  - Complete an incident report per facility policy
  - Confirm the chemical or biological indicator results
  - Inform appropriate leadership
  - Investigate the failure
  - Quarantine potentially affected items

Evaluate and Ensure

- Evaluate all packaging and containers to ensure integrity and sterilization before dispensing to the sterile field.
- Ensure the AORN guidelines for sterile processing are followed.
  - Sterilization processes include
    - Items sterilized in designated processing areas
    - Phacoemulsification handpieces in a vertical position
    - Reusable sterilized semi-critical items
  - Sterilization, instead of high-level disinfection, is considered more effective in the prevention of transmissible pathogens.

ALERT!

AORN recommends that healthcare organizations do the following:

- Designate only qualified individuals to manage and oversee sterile processing personnel.
- Increase awareness of the environmental impact of the sterilization process.
- Monitor and control the flow of steam to sterilizers.
- Standardize and monitor off-site sterilization processes.

- Ensure that all perioperative and sterile processing personnel.
    - Are aware of work hazards and handling of hazardous chemical sterilizers, including the following:
        - *Ethylene oxide*: A vapor or gas used to sterilize surgical items that are moisture- or heat-sensitive.
        - *Hydrogen peroxide*: A vapor or gas used to sterilize moisture- and heat-sensitive items.
        - *Peracetic acid*: A liquid chemical sterilant used for devices that can be immersed and cannot be sterilized using steam.
    - Know the IUSS process (formerly known as flash sterilization).
    - Follow instructions for rigid container use during the IUSS cycle and only use IUSS cycles when
        - Item is for immediate use
        - Terminal sterilization process is not possible
        - Device manufacturer provides written instructions for using IUSS related to cleaning, sterilization cycle type, exposure, temperature, and drying parameters.
    - Perform management processes for a wet pack or wet load, including the following:
        - Take corrective action when there is moisture on or in a package.
        - Reassess the entire load as moisture on or in a package possibly indicates problems with the sterilizer, steam supply, or load configuration.
        - Resterilize the package.
    - Process reusable medical devices based on how they are intended for use.
        - Devices that are labeled for single use only should not be reprocessed.
        - Surgical items that enter sterile tissues should be sterile when used.
    - Store sterile items in controlled conditions.
        - Determine the shelf life of sterilized items and purge expired items on a routine basis.
        - Remove all shipping containers and open-edged corrugated boxes before transfer to the OR/perioperative area.
    - Transport sterile items according to facility policy and with adherence to CDC, FDA, and AORN guidelines.
        - Protect sterile items from contamination, damage, or tampering during transport.
        - Transport sterile items using a sterile barrier system.
        - Use carts or bins that are covered and have solid bottoms.
    - Understand how to use MSDSs in the event of exposure.
    - Use a sterile barrier system to transport all sterile items to the point of use.
    - Use biological indicators specific to each sterilization process and type of sterilizer.
- Ensure that the instrumentation is returned to its original container or a transport container by
    - Disassembling all instruments with removable parts.
    - Flushing sterile water through hollow instruments.
    - Opening hinged instruments to expose box locks or serrated edges.
    - Separating delicate and small instruments with sharp edges.

UNFOLDING SCENARIO 7D

During the abdominal procedure, the circulating nurse opens the tray for the Bookwalter retractor set. Upon inspection, the nurse notes that the chemical indicator is missing. Only two of these retractor sets are available, and the other one is being used in another case. The surgeon wants the retractor set IUSS to use in this case.

Question

What is the nurse's next course of action?

DOCUMENTATION OF STERILIZATION AND DISINFECTION

The perioperative nurse verifies that documentation of sterilization and disinfection is complete for steam and high-level disinfection. This section reviews AORN's recommendations related to the documentation of sterilization processes.

Assess

- Assess the IUSS daily and upon each use for appropriate functioning according to the facility policy and procedures.
- Assess sterilization logs for accuracy and completeness.

Confirm

Confirm that the following documentation requirements are completed related to all methods of sterilization:
- Contents
- Exposure parameters
- Load number
- Operator's name or initials
- Results of physical, chemical, and biological monitors
- Sterilization records in compliance with the healthcare organization's policies and regulations at the federal, state, and local levels

Evaluate and Ensure

- Evaluate and ensure that perioperative or sterile processing personnel use physical monitors to ensure that every cycle meets appropriate high-level and steam sterilization parameters by verifying printouts, digital monitors, graphs, or gauges. High-level disinfection documentation requires that designated personnel complete the following:
  - Documentation to demonstrate compliance with local, state, and federal regulations and accrediting agency requirements
  - Ongoing documentation maintenance
- Evaluate documentation of the following components for each reprocessed medical device:
  - Date and time of high-level disinfection processing
  - Description of the medical device or item
  - Medical device identification number
  - Method of cleaning
  - Name and title of the person performing the high-level disinfection
  - Name of the patient on whom the device was used
  - Name of the surgeon or physician
  - Name of the procedure for which the medical device was used
  - Processing exposure time
  - Quantity of the medical devices, if appropriate to process more than one at a time
  - Solution temperature, lot number, expiration date, and solution test strip quality control as applicable
- Ensure that IUSS documentation includes document cycle information and monitoring results, including
  - Cycle parameters
  - Date and time of the cycle
  - Items processed
  - Monitoring results
  - Operator information
  - Patient identification
  - Reason for IUSS
  - Type of cycle

 ALERT!

The FDA has established rules that guide manufacturers in the information they provide health professionals on the care, treatment, use, and sterilization of materials and instruments used on patients. This information is known as Information for Use (manufacturer's recommendations).

UNFOLDING SCENARIO 7E

At the end of the abdominal case, the circulator wraps up documentation on the abdominal case. Part of the documentation includes logging IUSS for the Bookwalter retractor set. The nurse confirms that the date, instrument, and time are written in the log. At the end of the abdominal procedure, the scrub person is returning the instrumentation to the respective trays. The circulator notices that a blade was left on a knife handle in the tray.

Question

What other types of information should the nurse be sure to document? What should the circulator do regarding the blade left on the knife handle?

TRACKING OF MATERIALS AND INSTRUMENTS

- Tracking of materials and instruments for use in the surgical setting consists of adherence to the manufacturer's recommendations for handling and use in surgery.
- Streamlining instrument sets promotes ease of tracking and encourages the preparation of trays that have a safe weight limit, the identification of limited quantity sets, and the identification of specialty-specific instrumentation.
- This section reviews the handling of materials and instruments, IFU guidance, and regulations associated with tracking.

Assess

Assess that the perioperative nurse and the sterile processing staff are using tracking processes and facility-approved systems for instrumentation and materials according to facility policy, including instruments and devices that are new to the facility, on loan, refurbished, or repaired.

- If a facility uses a scanning system, the nurse should scan the cart as outlined in the facility's policies and procedures.
- If the facility uses a manual checking process, the nurse should adhere to the process to ensure that the contents of the cart for each case have been accounted for and to prevent delays.

Confirm

Confirm that the tracking of materials and instruments follows:
- Facility policy and AORN recommendations
- FDA standards, including
  - Approval of the instrument and device usage in surgery
  - Review of the manufacturer's written instructions on proper cleaning and decontamination methods for the instrument and device

Evaluate and Ensure

- Evaluate surgical cases in advance and ensure that materials and instrumentation are received in the facility before the intended surgery to allow for standard terminal sterilization.
- Evaluate all instrumentation for
  - Ability to be powered on and off
  - Abnormalities associated with rough edges
  - Cleanliness
  - Completeness
  - Correct alignment
  - Corrosion, pitting, burrs, and cracks

ALERT!

TJC indicates that IUSS does not replace standard terminal sterilization and should not be used for convenience.

(continued)

Evaluate and Ensure *(continued)*

- Integrity of cords and insulation
- Retained moisture
- Ensure that perioperative and sterile processing personnel follow the manufacturer's IFU to
  - Avoid having to use IUSS
  - Address the use of reprocessing for single-use devices and register with the FDA
  - Decontaminate properly before return to the vendor
  - Handle single-use devices
  - Perform sterilization processes associated with cleaning, decontaminating, high-level disinfecting, inspection, and sterilization
- Ensure that the use of instrument and material tracking software, processes, or tools is performed according to facility policy and procedure.
- Ensure that all patient adverse events that cause harm, injury, or death are reported per facility policy and that the following FDA guidance is followed related to devices that have caused harm.
  - FDA can issue a tracking order for any specific device known to cause harm.
  - Use a formal tracking mechanism for any reprocessed instrument that has been recalled.

 POP QUIZ 7.1

The circulator begins a review of the case cart for the next case using the preference list taped to the top of the cart. The facility uses a barcode scanning system for all case carts. The circulator is in a hurry and does not scan the cart. Why is this a problem?

ENVIRONMENTAL CLEANING

Environmental cleaning is the process of cleaning, disinfecting, and monitoring the environment for cleanliness. Pathogen persistence on inanimate surfaces is as follows:
- *Escherichia coli*: 1.5 hr to 16 months
- *Enterococcus faecalis*: 5 days to 4 months
- *Pseudomonas aeruginosa*: 6 hr to 16 months
- *Staphylococcus aureus*: 7 days to 7 months

Assess

Assess all areas of the surgical suite for cleanliness before opening sterile contents for the case.

Confirm

Confirm that cleaning procedures avoid the use of the following:
- Brooms with bristles to sweep the floor in semi-restricted or restricted areas
- Dry mops
- Items that may cause aerosolization of particulates in the air
- Self-dispensing chemical spray mops
- Spray bottles for environmental surface disinfectants

Evaluate and Ensure

Evaluate and ensure that perioperative and sterile processing personnel have cleaned high-touch areas as follows:
- Preliminary cleaning before the first case of the day
  - Damp dust all horizontal surfaces in OR/procedure rooms with facility-approved disinfectants.
- Interim cleaning between cases
  - Clean all flat surfaces and surfaces that made contact with the patient.
  - Mop floors with damp or wet mops.

- Enhanced cleaning
  - Occurs when patients are infected with an MDRO or when specific pathogens are present, such as
    - *C. difficile*
    - CJD
    - MRSA
    - TB
- Terminal cleaning in all areas daily
  - Clean all surfaces, including wheels and casters.
  - Clean floors with a wet mop.
  - Wipe down walls, ceilings, sterile storage areas, equipment rooms, ice machines, and sink.

POP QUIZ 7.2

What should the circulator do in the surgical suite before bringing the case cart in for the next case?

ENVIRONMENTAL CONDITIONS OF THE STERILIZATION AND STORAGE AREAS

- Maintain environmental conditions and preserve the integrity of sterilized materials and instrumentation by managing humidity, temperature, moisture, and dust; heating and air ventilation systems; exposure to direct sunlight; and storage of materials and instrumentation. Limit the flow of traffic and movement around sterilized products.
- Perioperative personnel should monitor the thermostat and humidity and notify designated personnel to mitigate any issue related to heating, ventilating, and air conditioning.

Assess

Assess the surgical suite for the recommended environmental control settings as follows:
- Perioperative suite
  - Humidity 20% to 60%
  - Positive pressure ventilation system
  - Temperature 68 °F to 75 °F (20 °C–24 °C)
- Sterile processing cleanroom
  - Humidity maximum 60%
  - Positive pressure ventilation system
  - Temperature 68 °F to 73 °F (20 °C–23 °C)
- Endoscopy suite
  - Humidity 20% to 60%
  - Negative pressure for decontamination area
  - Temperature 68 °F to 73 °F (20 °C–23 °C)
- Procedure room
  - Humidity 20% to 60%
  - Positive pressure ventilation system
  - Temperature 68 °F to 73 °F (20 °C–23 °C)
- Sterile storage
  - Humidity maximum 60%
  - Positive pressure ventilation system
  - Temperature maximum 75 °F (24 °C)

Confirm

Confirm the following is performed related to the storage of sterilized products by perioperative and sterile processing personnel:
- Avoid dragging wrapped material to prevent tearing of wrapping.
- Use dust covers when appropriate.
- Follow hand hygiene and surgical attire practices per facility policies.
- Ensure shelving is free from damage or burrs that could damage packaging.

(continued)

Confirm *(continued)*

- Configure shelving and space to ensure adequate air circulation from all angles.
- Ensure that stacking occurs per the manufacturer's IFU.

Evaluate and Ensure

- Evaluate and ensure that traffic and movement are limited in relation to stored sterilized materials and instrumentation.
- Ensure CDC and AORN guidelines are followed related to the storage of sterile materials and instrumentation:
  - Date every sterilized product.
  - Monitor sterility of all sterile products on a routine basis.
  - Store sterile supplies and instruments in areas free from moisture, such as in closed cabinets or covered racks.
  - Store sterile supplies 8 to 10 in. from the floor, 5 in. from the ceiling, 18 in. from a sprinkler head, and 2 in. from an outside wall.
  - Use the facility-approved shelf-life practice for evaluating sterile materials (i.e., event related or time related).

HANDLING OF HAZARDOUS AND BIOHAZARDOUS MATERIALS

The perioperative nurse works to reduce risks associated with selecting, transporting, handling, and disposing of hazardous materials. Hazardous materials include those that cause radiation exposure, chemical exposure, or blood-borne pathogen exposure.

Assess

- Assess the risks associated with handling hazardous and biohazardous materials for each case.
- Assess the surgical suite for the presence of
  - Adequate PPE supply
  - Correct distance from the surgical suite to the nearest eyewash station and scrub sink
  - Supplies to confine and contain biohazardous fluid spills

Confirm

- Confirm that all perioperative personnel and visitors work to minimize radiation exposure by
  - Maintaining a distance of 6 ft. from the radiation source
  - Remaining behind leaded shielding when ionizing radiation use occurs
  - Protecting the patient with appropriate lead shielding
  - Wearing protective lead and moving as far as possible away from the source while maintaining aseptic technique for scrubbed personnel
- Confirm that perioperative personnel reports biohazardous exposures (blood, bodily fluids, chemicals, and radiation) to the employer per OSHA guidelines.

Evaluate and Ensure

- Evaluate the need for the following protective equipment and ensure its use by all personnel and when appropriate for the patient within the surgical suite when radiation exposure is likely
  - Flexible leaded aprons
  - Lead vests, skirts, thyroid shields, and gloves
  - Leaded safety eyeglasses with side shields
  - PPE for radioactive chemicals and drugs
  - Rigid shields on wheels

- Ensure that all members of the perioperative team don the appropriate PPE to protect against blood-borne pathogen transmission through the following:
  - Debris: Tissue or blood on instrumentation, sharps, and needlesticks
  - Fluids: Cerebrospinal fluid, synovial fluid, pleural fluid, peritoneal fluid, and amniotic fluid
  - Secretions: Semen, vaginal discharge, saliva, and mucous
  - Tissue: Central nervous system tissue
- Ensure hand hygiene is performed after the following occurs:
  - Patient contact
  - Removal of gloves
  - Touching blood or body fluids
  - Touching contaminated items
- Ensure compliance with OSHA blood-borne pathogens standards relating to reducing exposure to blood, bodily fluids, and infectious or hazardous materials.
  - Attend training on the prevention of occupational exposure to blood, bodily fluids, and hazardous chemicals.
  - Restrict the activities of personnel who have infections, open lesions, or nonintact skin.
  - Use safety devices, neutral zones, and hands-free techniques to reduce exposure to sharps injuries.
  - Wear PPE at all times.
- Ensure that infectious and noninfectious tissues and waste are managed according to OSHA and AORN's position statement for environmental responsibility.
  - Eliminate mercury-based products.
  - Follow the waste removal protocols established by the organization related to recycling, disposal, dilution, or deactivation (i.e., radioactive or other chemical fluids).
  - Limit the use of biohazardous waste containers to infectious waste (i.e., red bag).
  - Survey the type of waste that is projected to be produced by the procedure and plan availability of requisite equipment and supplies for potential spillage and collection.
  - Use a bag-in-bag collection system to reduce the risks to healthcare workers.

> ### 🔊 ALERT!
>
> When managing a case associated with CJD, which is a fatal neurodegenerative disease:
>
> - Use disposable instrumentation sets for diagnostic brain biopsies to rule out CJD or TSE.
> - Do not use chemical or physical methods, including steam autoclaving, dry heat, or ethylene oxide gas. Chemical disinfection with formaldehyde or glutaraldehyde will destroy the prions that cause the disease.

> ### POP QUIZ 7.3
>
> The circulating nurse is preparing for a patient scheduled to undergo an open reduction internal fixation of the left ankle. The nurse opens a tray of instruments and discovers moisture. What is the appropriate next step?

RESOURCES

Association for periOperative Registered Nurses. (2019). *Guideline essentials: Key takeaways. Sterilization.* https://www.aorn.org/essentials/sterilization

Association for periOperative Registered Nurses. (2020a). AORN position statement on environmental responsibility. *AORN Journal, 111*(6), 1–11. https://doi.org/10.1002/aorn.13063

Association for periOperative Registered Nurses. (2020b). *Guideline essentials: Key takeaways. Environmental cleaning.* https://www.aorn.org/essentials/environmental-cleaning

Association for periOperative Registered Nurses. (2020c). *Guideline essentials: Key takeaways. Packaging.* https://www.aorn.org/essentials/packaging-systems

Association for periOperative Registered Nurses. (2021a). *Guideline for design and maintenance, Guidelines for perioperative practice.* Author.

Association for periOperative Registered Nurses. (2021b). *Guideline for environmental cleaning, Guidelines for perioperative practice*. Author.

Association for periOperative Registered Nurses. (2021c). *Guideline for environment of care, Guidelines for perioperative practice*. Author.

Association for periOperative Registered Nurses. (2021d). *Guideline for hand hygiene, Guidelines for perioperative practice*. Author.

Association for periOperative Registered Nurses. (2021e). *Guideline for high level disinfection, Guidelines for perioperative practice*. Author.

Association for periOperative Registered Nurses. (2021f). *Guideline for instrument cleaning, Guidelines for perioperative practice*. Author.

Association for periOperative Registered Nurses. (2021g). *Guideline for packaging systems, Guidelines for perioperative practice*. Author.

Association for periOperative Registered Nurses. (2021h). *Guideline for radiation safety, Guidelines for perioperative practice*. Author.

Association for periOperative Registered Nurses. (2021i). *Guideline for sharps safety, Guidelines for perioperative practice*. Author.

Association for periOperative Registered Nurses. (2021j). *Guideline for sterile technique, Guidelines for perioperative practice*. Author.

Association for periOperative Registered Nurses. (2021k). *Guideline for sterilization, Guidelines for perioperative practice*. Author.

Association for periOperative Registered Nurses. (2021l). *Guideline for surgical attire, Guidelines for perioperative practice*. Author.

Berríos-Torres, S. I., Umscheid, C. A., Bratzler, D. W., Leas, B., Stone, E. C., Kelz, R. R., Reinke, C. E., Morgan, S., Solomkin, J. S., Mazuski, J. E., Dellinger, E. P., Itani, K. M. F., Berbari, E. F., Segreti, J., Parvizi, J., Blanchard, J., Allen, G., Kluytmans, J. A. J. W., . . . Donlan, R. (2017). Centers for disease control and prevention guideline for the prevention of surgical site infection, 2017. *JAMA Surgery, 152*(8), 784–791. https://www.cdc.gov/infection control/guidelines/ssi/index.html

Centers for Disease Control and Prevention. (2016a). *Standard precautions for all patient care*. U.S. Department of Health and Human Services, Centers for Disease Control and Prevention. https://www.cdc.gov/infection control/basics/standard-precautions.html

Centers for Disease Control and Prevention. (2016b). *Transmission-based precautions*. U.S. Department of Health and Human Services, Centers for Disease Control and Prevention. https://www.cdc.gov/infectioncontrol/basics/transmission-based-precautions.html

The Joint Commission. (2013). *The Joint Commission's implementation guide for NPSG.07.05.01 on surgical site infections: The SSI change project*. https://www.jointcommission.org/-/media/tjc/documents/resources/hai/implementation_guide_for_npsg_ssipdf.pdf

The Joint Commission. (2021a, January 1). *Hospital: 2021 national patient safety goals*. https://www.joint commission.org/standards/national-patient-safety-goals/hospital-national-patient-safety-goals/

The Joint Commission. (2021b, March 1). *Instrument reprocessing—Immediate use steam sterilization (IUSS): What are important considerations associated with immediate-use steam sterilization?* https://www.jointcommission.org/standards/standard-faqs/ambulatory/infection-prevention-and-control-ic/000002122/

The Joint Commission. (n.d). *Surgical site infections*. https://www.jointcommission.org/resources/patient-safety-topics/infection-prevention-and-control/surgical-site-infections/

Occupational Safety and Health Administration. (n.d.-a). *Bloodborne pathogens and needlestick prevention*. United States Department of Labor, Occupational Safety and Health Administration. https://www.osha.gov/blood borne-pathogens/standards

Occupational Safety and Health Administration. (n.d.-b). *Personal protective equipment*. United States Department of Labor, Occupational Safety and Health Administration. https://www.osha.gov/personal-protective-equipment

Rothrock, J. C. (2019). *Alexander's care of the patient in surgery* (16th ed.). Elsevier—Health Sciences Division.

8

EMERGENCY SITUATIONS

OVERVIEW

- Emergency situations can arise at any time in the perioperative suite. This chapter reviews some of the most common emergent situations, including the following:
  - Anaphylaxis
  - Conversion to an open procedure
  - Difficult airway
  - Environmental hazards
  - Hemorrhage
  - LAST
  - MH
  - Mass casualty, triage, and evacuation
  - Perioperative cardiac arrest
  - Trauma
- Throughout each phase of the perioperative experience, the nurse will perform duties using the ACE process:
  - Assess
  - Confirm
  - Evaluate and Ensure

ANAPHYLAXIS

Anaphylaxis is a type I hypersensitivity reaction and medical emergency that occurs in response to exposure to an allergen. The occurrence of anaphylaxis in the OR is rare. It is primarily related to latex exposure associated with products used for patient handling and the procedure, neuromuscular blocking drugs, or antibiotic allergies that are unknown to the patient.

Assess

- Assess the patient and family history for allergic reactions to the following:
  - Antibiotics
  - Induction medications
  - Intraoperative medications and fluorescent dyes (hyaluronidase, methylene blue, coagulation agents, trypan blue, indocyanine green, and colloids)
  - Latex
  - Neuromuscular blocking drugs
  - Skin prepping agents (chlorhexidine, betadine, and alcohol)
- Assess the patient for risk factors associated with latex sensitivity, such as
  - Food allergies (banana, kiwi, avocado, chestnut, and raw potato)
  - History of long-term bladder care, spina bifida, spinal cord trauma, urogenital abnormalities, or multiple procedures
  - Symptoms associated with asthma, dermatitis, urticaria, hay fever, or rhinitis

Table 8.1 Signs and Symptoms of Anaphylactic Reactions

Body System	Signs and Symptoms
Cardiovascular	Tachycardia, hypotension, arrhythmias
Genitourinary	Reduced urine output
Hematologic	DIC
Integumentary	Urticaria, pruritis, edema, erythema
Respiratory	Dyspnea, hypoxia, pulmonary edema, bronchospasm, increased respirations

Assess *(continued)*
- Assess the patient for signs and symptoms of anaphylactic reactions. Table 8.1 lists common signs and symptoms.
- Assess the patient's skin postoperatively for signs and symptoms of dermatitis, erythema, edema, or impaired skin integrity.

Confirm

Confirm the following:
- All drugs used during the procedure are verified with the surgeon and anesthesia personnel before dispensing to the field.
- Epinephrine is available and ready for use on the patient during the emergency.
- Patient-reported allergies are shared with all members of the surgical team.
- The causative agent and associated products are discontinued and removed rapidly upon patient presentation with anaphylaxis.

 ALERT!

For patients with known latex allergy, remove all items that might contain latex, such as gloves, catheters, IV equipment, tape, tourniquets, ventilation and airway equipment, and medication stoppers.

Evaluate and Ensure

- Ensure the following have been completed intraoperatively and in preparation for an anaphylactic reaction:
  - Confirmation that medications that will serve to counteract the reaction (epinephrine, vasopressin, diphenhydramine, ranitidine, famotidine, hydrocortisone, methylprednisolone, and albuterol) are available
  - Confirmation that low-protein and powder-free gloves are available
  - Latex precautions for patients with known latex sensitivity or allergy
  - Presence of the code cart and defibrillator in the surgical suite
  - Protection of the sterile field by the scrub person during the emergency

 NURSING PEARL

Use the **ALLERGIC** mnemonic to remember how to proactively protect the patient from an allergic reaction:
- **A**ssess the patient for known allergies
- **L**atex products must be removed if a problem
- **L**imit the traffic in the suite
- **E**pinephrine bolus and fluids should be available
- **R**escue drugs and code cart should be available
- **G**love selection should be appropriate based on patient allergies
- **I**solate and protect the sterile field
- **C**ausative agents should be identified

- Restriction of traffic in the surgical suite
- Placement of signs and patient armbands for patients who have a latex or medication allergy
- Evaluate the code cart to ensure that the contents have been checked according to facility policy and the defibrillator is operational.

CONVERSION TO AN OPEN PROCEDURE

- Conversion to an open procedure can occur with laparoscopic and robotic surgical approaches.
- Conversion is considered an emergent situation and will occur when complications arise, including the following:
  - Bleeding or hemorrhage from a puncture, tissue cuts and tears, suture or surgical clip failure, or other vessel disruption
  - Gas embolism, which can cause cardiovascular collapse
  - Hypothermia from carbon dioxide insufflation colder than the body temperature of the patient
  - Incidental iatrogenic injury from positioning aids, port placement, surgical errors, robotic attachments, or placement of other equipment
  - Perforation of a major organ or vessel related to trocars and rigid scopes used during surgery
  - Preperitoneal insufflation from gas that has not been evacuated using the inlet side port, which occurs when a trocar instead of a Veress needle is used to insufflate.

Assess

- Assess for potential anesthesia factors that could contribute to conversion to an open procedure from either laparoscopic or robotic surgical procedure, such as
  - Inadequate muscle relaxation for the procedure
  - Ineffective hemodynamic stability
  - Respiratory instability associated with insufflation and hypoxia
- Assess for surgical factors that can contribute to conversion to an open procedure from either laparoscopic or robotic surgical procedure, such as
  - Hemorrhage related to surgical error or change in patient's status
  - Manipulation of the robot master controls
  - Placement of ports
  - Skill set related to the use of the robotic system or laparoscopic trocars and instruments
  - Testing of systems related to laparoscopic or robotic procedures (insufflation, electrocautery unit, foot pedals and connections, video tower and power sources, etc.)

 POP QUIZ 8.1

A 42-year-old nulliparous female presents to the OR for a bilateral breast mastectomy related to the finding of breast cancer in both breasts. She has a medical history of hypertension and DM. Both conditions are well controlled. During the preoperative assessment, the patient reports having an allergic reaction to penicillin, which causes a rash. This is the patient's first surgical procedure. The surgeon indicates that she will also perform sentinel node biopsy and lymphatic mapping and asks that isosulfan blue dye be dispensed to the surgical field. The patient will be administered general anesthesia.

During the procedure, the surgeon begins the lymphatic mapping and injects the isosulfan blue dye. The anesthesiologist alerts the surgeon that the patient's blood pressure has dropped to 62/40 and her heart rate has spiked to 125 bpm. The patient also exhibits labored breathing. What is happening to the patient, and what should the circulating nurse do next?

 NURSING PEARL

Use the **CONVERT** mnemonic to use when converting to an open procedure from a laparoscopic procedure and when the risk of hemorrhage is evident:

- **C**all for help
- **O**pen additional supplies as needed
- **N**otify the blood bank
- **V**erify blood products
- **E**mergency code cart should be obtained
- **R**emove all contents from the surgical wound and perform a count when feasible
- **T**urn all lights on and turn off the fiber optic light source to prevent fire

(continued)

Assess *(continued)*

- Assess for potential technical factors that can contribute to conversion to an open procedure from either a laparoscopic or robotic surgical procedure, such as
  - Technical issues related to equipment or instrumentation
  - Video imaging issues that cause insufficient visibility
- Assess the consent and ensure that the potential to convert to an open procedure is written on the consent.

Confirm

- Confirm that the following have been performed related to conversion to an open procedure from the robotic or laparoscopic procedure:
  - Complete a full count of all instrumentation, sharps, and sponges at the beginning of the procedure in preparation for potential conversion.
  - Follow facility policy on the need to perform a second time-out for robotic procedures during which each member of the team verbalizes what should be done in the event of conversion to an open procedure.
  - Notify or page additional surgeons as requested by the attending surgeon.
  - Open additional instrumentation, sharps, and sponges as needed.
  - Safely disconnect all cords attached to the equipment for lights, ultrasonic, and other power sources that will not be used during the open procedure.
  - Turn on the overhead lights and OR lights.
  - Undock the robot.

Evaluate and Ensure

- Evaluate the type of emergency associated with the procedure (technical, surgical, or anesthetic).
- Evaluate the patient assessment performed by the surgeon and confer with the surgical team on the reasons conversion to an open procedure might occur, such as
  - Distorted anatomy that would inhibit safe dissection
  - Gross contamination or infection within a cavity
  - Hemorrhage
  - Patient's intolerance to pneumoperitoneum or the required positioning or concerns raised by the anesthesia personnel related to the inability to provide safe respiratory support
  - Presence of abdominal adhesions
- Ensure that the patient is prepped and draped in a manner that will preserve sterility at the field and in preparation for potential conversion to open procedure.
- Ensure that the time of conversion and any changes in patient status are recorded in the nursing documentation.

 POP QUIZ 8.2

A 62-year-old patient presents to the OR suite for laparoscopic cholecystectomy. The patient is positioned, intubated, draped, and prepped. The time-out is performed. The surgical incision has been made, and the first port is placed using the Hassan technique. Insufflation of the abdominal cavity has commenced. The surgeon introduces the laparoscope with the RN first assistant standing by to place the next port. When the surgeon advances the laparoscope, it shows multiple adhesions wrapped around the liver and adjacent organs. The surgeon notes that the gall bladder is oozing due to pressure from the adhesions. The surgeon alerts the anesthesiologist that the case will need to convert to an open procedure. The anesthesiologist begins to stabilize the patient for the change in position. The surgeon begins to decompress the abdomen and release the gas. What is the role of the circulating nurse in this scenario?

DIFFICULT AIRWAY

There are times when a patient presents to the OR suite with a difficult airway related to a medical emergency, the patient's medical and surgical history, or congenital or acquired anatomic defects of the airway. The presentation of a difficult airway is often unanticipated and creates challenges for the anesthesia team related to airway management. Although the management of the patient's airway falls under the scope of practice for anesthesia personnel, the perioperative nurse must provide support to the patient and the anesthesia team by being present at the bedside during induction and emergence.

Assess

- Assess the patient's medical history associated with
  - Congenital or acquired anatomic defects
  - History of facial, neck, or chest trauma
  - History of regurgitation, obesity, or oral cavity disease

Confirm

- Confirm availability of the airway management supplies.
- Confirm that the patient is in the appropriate position to maximize exposure for intubation.

Evaluate and Ensure

- Evaluate the patient's response to activities occurring within the sterile field throughout the entire procedure.
- Ensure the following associated with patient safety:
  - Patient is positioned so that the head is in neutral alignment with the vertebral axis, the cervical spine is stable, and the head is slightly extended.
  - Support is provided to the anesthesia team by remaining at the head of the bed and providing necessary assistance related to the application of cricoid pressure, inflation of the cuff, or removal of the stylet.
  - The safety strap is securely placed in an area that maximizes exposure to the surgical site and does not constrict breathing.

NURSING PEARL

The ASA defines a *difficult airway* as a "clinical situation wherein a trained anesthesiologist cannot achieve effective facemask ventilation of the upper airway, establish tracheal intubation, or both."

POP QUIZ 8.3

A 65-year-old man presents to the OR suite directly from the emergency room with a possible ruptured appendix. The report from the emergency room physician indicates that the patient said he had been vomiting, has had diarrhea for over 24 hr, and is experiencing intense pain in the right lower abdomen. During induction, the anesthesiologist reports that intubation through direct laryngoscopy is difficult. The nurse anesthetist retrieves the difficult airway cart. What is the role of the perioperative circulating nurse?

ENVIRONMENTAL HAZARD EMERGENCIES

- The perioperative nurse must work with the surgical team to mitigate the risks associated with environmental hazards in and around the surgical suite. Environmental hazards in the surgical suite include the following:
  - Blood-borne pathogens and hazardous waste
  - Chemical exposure
  - Compressed gases
  - Communicable disease exposure
  - Equipment burns or shocks
  - Fire
  - Laser use
  - Radiation exposure
  - Slips, trips, and falls
  - Smoke plume
  - Waste anesthetic gases

Assess

Assess the surgical suite continuously for potential environmental hazards.

Confirm

The perioperative nurse should confirm with the surgical team that the potential for occupational injury from exposure to harmful chemicals, waste, and pathogens has been evaluated and voice any concerns before the start of a procedure.

Evaluate and Ensure

Evaluate for and ensure that actions are taken to mitigate injury associated with environmental hazards. Table 8.2 lists common environmental hazards and associated nursing actions.

 NURSING PEARL

Working to prevent injury in the work environment is essential. Benjamin Franklin once said, "An ounce of prevention is worth a pound of cure."

 POP QUIZ 8.4

The OR suite has been prepped for a right shoulder arthroscopy with rotator cuff repair. As the procedure commences, the perioperative circulating nurse performs a safety evaluation. The nurse notes that multiple cords and equipment affect the traffic pattern in the surgical suite. What is the best course of action for the nurse to take to ensure safety?

Table 8.2 Environmental Hazards and Actions

Hazards	Actions
Blood-borne pathogens and hazardous waste	• Routinely replace all sharps containers to ensure there is a means for disposing of sharps safely. • Ensure all staff are wearing appropriate personal protective equipment in anticipation of exposure to blood-borne pathogens, chemicals, and laser use. • Promote the use of double-gloving, blunted needles, and safe zones for the passing of sharps.
Chemical exposure	• Handle and store all chemicals according to the manufacturer's recommendation and MSDS (disinfectants, sterilants, tissue preservatives, antiseptic agents). • Educate staff on the use of eyewash stations based on facility policy. • Ensure eyewash stations are plumbed or self-contained and in close proximity to where chemicals are handled. • Review emergency spill plans and respiratory protection plans with staff and keep copies in an area in close proximity to where chemicals are handled.
Communicable disease exposure	• Follow facility, state, local, and federal guidelines associated with identification, isolation, and treatment of patients with communicable diseases (tuberculosis, HIV/AIDS, etc.). • Maintain personal protective equipment (PPE) protocols associated with the organism. • Maintain the appropriate air exchanges associated with caring for a patient with a communicable disease. • Reduce airborne particle spread by restricting traffic within the suite.
Compressed gases	• Check cylinders before use for evidence of the appropriate labeling, color-coding, and pin safety according to facility policy. • Store an emergency supply of oxygen according to facility policy. • Store medical gases in a secured location away from industrial gases and routes of egress. • Transport medical gases in facility-approved carriers that are designed to prevent cylinders from being dropped or tipped. • Use approved fittings, flow control devices, and regulators associated with the medical gas.

(continued)

Table 8.2 Environmental Hazards and Actions *(continued)*

Hazards	Actions
Equipment burns or shocks	• Inspect all electrical equipment for damage and integrity of the cord insulation. • Remove equipment with frayed cords or damage and report per facility procedure. • Use devices according to manufacturers' guidelines.
Fire	• Perform a fire safety assessment before each case associated with ignition sources, fuels, and the potential for an oxygen-enriched environment. • Prevent contact between fuels (e.g., alcohol-based skin antiseptic agents, drapes, and gowns) and ignition sources. • Use ignition sources according to manufacturer's guidelines (e.g., electrosurgical electrodes, fiber-optic light cords).
Laser use	• Attach extra laser protective eyewear to the door with a sign. • Cover windows in the nominal hazard zone with a barrier that blocks the laser beam. • Display warning signs on each door of the surgical suite. • Ensure that the laser has been maintained and checked by facility-authorized technicians. • Limit the traffic in the suite to those who are trained in laser safety precautions. • Perform appropriate calibration of the beam before each procedure. • Perform a laser-safety time-out before the start of the laser procedure. • Place laser in standby mode when not in use. • Use appropriate filters or barriers according to OSHA standards. • Use laser protective eyewear.
Radiation exposure	• Protect the patient from radiation exposure by applying the appropriate lead shield after the patient has been positioned for surgery. • Wear a passive dosimeter to monitor personal radiation exposure associated with x-ray equipment and radioactive patients or materials. • Wear appropriate lead aprons, gloves, thyroid shields, and goggles when in contact with radiation.
Slips, trips, and falls	• Arrange equipment and supplies so that the suite is not cluttered, and pathways are not obstructed. • Cover electrical cables on the floor with a facility-approved cord cover. • Provide appropriate lighting within the suite. • Post signs where wet floor hazards exist. • Rapidly clean up spills or debris. • Wear slip-resistant shoes or facility-approved shoe covers.
Smoke plume	• Treat all tubing, filters, and absorbers as infectious waste. • Routinely inspect smoke evacuation equipment for proper functioning. • Use smoke evacuation equipment and inline suction filters for each case.
Waste anesthetic gases	• Provide enough ventilation to keep the room concentration of waste anesthetic gases below occupational exposure levels. • Report issues with ventilation and air exchanges promptly to the manager.

HEMORRHAGE

• With surgical intervention comes the risk of blood loss associated with hemorrhage due to medical error or anatomic dysfunction. DIC is associated with hemorrhage and is also a complication in surgery. *DIC* is an acquired systemic disorder that involves a combination of hemorrhage and microvascular coagulation. Hemorrhage and DIC are unexpected medical emergencies that can occur in the OR.

Assess

- Assess laboratory test data for prolonged bleeding times (i.e., PT, aPTT, and INR values).
- Assess the patient's medical and surgical history for previous issues with tissue healing.

Confirm

- Confirm that the patient has had a blood type, cross, and screen in preparation for planned blood loss during the procedure.
- Confirm availability of blood products with the laboratory.

Evaluate and Ensure

- Evaluate for signs and symptoms of DIC (e.g., profuse bleeding at the surgical site, petechiae).
- Ensure the following is addressed related to blood transfusion:
  - A two-person confirmation of blood products and patient identification is performed
  - Blood products are handled safely, and standard PPE is used
  - Blood products are used within the timeframe indicated by the facility and in accordance with the American Association of Blood Blanks guidelines
  - Transfusion reactions are noted in the perioperative record
- Ensure the following are addressed related to emergencies associated with perioperative hemorrhage:
  - Off the field
    - Dispense medications and other medical supplies as ordered by the surgeon in a timely fashion.
    - Provide support to anesthesia personnel related to the acquisition of blood products as needed.
  - On the field
    - Remove all sharps and other surgical products from the surgical field and account for all while the surgeon works to find the source of the bleeding.

POP QUIZ 8.5

A 47-year-old male is undergoing a laparoscopic cholecystectomy that requires emergent conversion to open procedure because the cystic artery is cut. The surgeon states that the patient is hemorrhaging. What should the circulating nurse do to assist in this situation?

LOCAL ANESTHETIC SYSTEMIC TOXICITY

- *LAST* is a life-threatening adverse event that involves the central nervous system and may be caused by the rate of absorption at the injection site, the injection technique, the type of anesthetic used, and/or patient characteristics.

Assess

- Assess patient characteristics that may increase the risk of LAST, such as
  - Disease processes associated with the liver, heart, pregnancy, and metabolic syndromes
  - Extremes of age
  - Known cardiac conduction or electrolyte abnormality
  - Low body mass index

Confirm

Confirm the dosage and route of the local injection with the surgeon.

Evaluate and Ensure

- Evaluate the patient for the following from 30 seconds to 60 minutes following injection:
  - EKG monitoring
    - Asystole
    - Bradycardia

NURSING PEARL

The LAST rescue kit should include a lipid emulsion 20%, large syringes (50 mL), IV administration supplies, and the American Society of Regional Anesthesia checklist. See Resources section for list details.

- ○ Ventricular fibrillation
- ○ Wide-QRS complex ventricular tachycardia
- Symptoms
  - ○ Confusion or disorientation
  - ○ Dizziness
  - ○ Drowsiness
  - ○ Local tissue response
  - ○ Metallic taste
  - ○ Oral numbness
- Ensure the following is completed if LAST is suspected:
  - Assist with administration of 20% lipid emulsion therapy
  - Assist with resuscitation
  - Call for help (code team, anesthesia personnel)
  - Establish or assist with IV access
  - Maintain the airway
  - Stop the administration of the local anesthetic
  - Ventilate with 100% oxygen

POP QUIZ 8.6

A 61-year-old male is admitted to the perioperative suite for an excision of a lipoma on the right leg. He has a low body mass index and atrial fibrillation. His past surgical history includes a bilateral inguinal hernia repair and a laparoscopic appendectomy. He reports having no adverse effects to anesthesia during past surgeries. At the start of the procedure, the surgeon requests that 0.5% bupivacaine and 1% lidocaine be dispensed to the sterile field for local injection. The surgeon injects 10 mL of lidocaine combined with 2 mL of bupivacaine at the start of the procedure. Five minutes after the injection, the patient displays confusion, says that his mouth feels numb, and becomes bradycardic. What should the circulating nurse do in response to the change in the patient's condition?

MALIGNANT HYPERTHERMIA

MH is an inherited pharmacogenetic syndrome that is caused by anesthetic agents and succinylcholine. The occurrence of MH in the operating suite is a life-threatening adverse event requiring swift action of the entire perioperative team to avert the progression of the crisis and patient death. The anesthesia team will alert the surgeon that an MH crisis is apparent, at which time the surgical procedure will come to a halt and life-saving measures will ensue.

Assess

Assess the patient's medical record related to the following:
- Allergies to medications or foods
- Anxiety and pain level
- Assistive devices
- Current medications
- Implanted devices
- Medical and surgical history
- Previous anesthesia complications

Confirm

- In known cases of complications associated with anesthesia, the nurse should confirm that the triggering agents are removed from the anesthesia workstation.
- The nurse should also confirm that the anesthetic agent has been properly flushed from the system and that all delivery lines and suction are new.
- The nurse should confirm that the MH cart is available.

Evaluate and Ensure

- Evaluate for any changes in the patient's status throughout the procedure.

NURSING PEARL

STOP what you are doing in an MH crisis:
- **S**top the volatile agents and succinylcholine.
- **T**reat the patient with supportive care, dantrolene, and cooling.
- **O**xygen *100%:* Use to flush out the volatile anesthetics.
- **P**repare to cool the patient with ice and IV saline.

(continued)

Evaluate and Ensure *(continued)*

- Ensure the following activities are completed during an MH crisis to assist anesthesia personnel:
  - Stop the use of volatile agents and succinylcholine.
  - Retrieve the following pharmacologic treatment products:
    - Calcium chloride (10%): A 10-mL vial, have two available
    - Dantrolene sodium: 2.5 mg/kg is recommended
    - Dextrose 50%: 50-mL vials, have two available
    - Lidocaine for injection (2%): 100 mg/5 mL or 100 mg/10 mL in preloaded syringes, have three available
    - Regular insulin: 100 units/mL, have one available but refrigerated
    - Refrigerated saline: At minimum 3,000 mL for IV cooling
    - Sodium bicarbonate (8.4%): 50-mL vials, have five available
    - Sterile water for injection United States Pharmacopeia (USP) (without a bacteriostatic agent): Available to reconstitute dantrolene
  - Retrieve the following nonpharmacologic treatments:
    - Ice lavage through the esophagus or rectal tube
    - Ice packs around the patient's body, head, and feet
  - Retrieve equipment/supplies that may be used during an MH crisis, including the following:
    - Activated charcoal filters
    - Blood gas kits
    - Central venous pressure kits (sizes appropriate to patient population)
    - Crushed ice and plastic bags
    - Esophageal and other core temperature probes
    - Syringes, needles, and transfer devices
    - Transducer kits for arterial and central venous cannulation
    - Urimeter
  - Report the crisis to the management team, MHAUS, and the PACU or ICU.
  - Report to MHAUS by calling the MHAUS Hotline (1-800-644-9737 or outside the U.S. 001-209-417-3722) for additional advice. A trained MH anesthesia person will join the anesthesiologist of record for the case to help to guide the crisis.

POP QUIZ 8.7

A healthy 17-year-old male is positioned for a right inguinal hernia repair. The patient has no prior surgical history. His parents report he has not had complications with anesthetic agents. Fifteen minutes into the surgery, the patient begins to exhibit signs and symptoms such as buccal rigidity, rapid heart rate, and decreased oxygen saturation rate. The anesthesiologist alerts the surgeon that the patient is experiencing MH. The surgeon stops the procedure and begins to close the wound. What should the perioperative circulating nurse initially do to assist the team?

MASS CASUALTY, TRIAGE, AND EVACUATION

- The perioperative nurse must be prepared to manage casualties caused by human-made and natural disasters.
- The facility policy for the management of casualty events and evacuation from the facility should be reviewed regularly to ensure that all staff are aware of the steps to take to triage patients, manage care, and prepare the OR to receive patients in an expedited manner.

Assess

- Assess the mass casualty event policy and plan to coordinate with the interprofessional team as well as outside agencies to coordinate patient care.
- Assess the population of patients and the resources needed to safely evacuate patients if a mass casualty event occurs in the healthcare facility.
- Assess the type of exposure or injuries expected (e.g., chemical, biological, radiological, nuclear, or incendiary incidents).

Confirm

- Confirm the following associated with the evacuation of patients:
  - Assembly of the patients according to ambulatory status, nonambulatory status, wheelchair-bound, mobility deficit, and critical care needs
  - When moving patients who have critical care needs
    - Perform a patient assessment of vital signs, IV lines, airway type and management needs, weight, and stability for transport.
    - Plan for the movement of equipment needed, consolidation of pumps, and emergency medications that may be needed during transport.
- Confirm the following associated with triaging patients:
  - Availability of resources needed for incoming cases
  - Use of the facility-approved system for prioritization of patients

Evaluate and Ensure

- Evaluate the supply lists generated for incoming cases and alert management if there will be any challenges or barriers related to the availability of products.
- Ensure that patients' needs are addressed in a timely fashion related to the level of triage, according to facility policy and AORN guidelines.
  - Critical or emergent requires surgical treatment of patients immediately.
  - Semi-critical requires surgical intervention within 6 to 8 hr.
- Ensure that the goals associated with surgical intervention in a mass casualty event are met, including the following:
  - Appropriate space available to assess and triage patients
  - Availability of blood and blood products
  - Availability of necessary equipment, instrumentation, and other medical supplies
  - Documentation of all interventions and barriers to providing care
  - Identification of team members who are skilled and trained to perform
  - Reduction in delays through efficient use of resources and time
  - Saving the most lives
  - Use of AORN standards and facility policy
- Ensure the following is addressed related to facility-wide evacuation:
  - Documentation of all patients and personnel evacuated
  - Effective communication between facilities and team personnel
  - Identification of patient's needs during the transfer of care
  - Mode of transportation
  - Preparation of patient's medical records and medications
  - Routes of egress and types of evacuation
    - Horizontal evacuation requires the movement of patients to the safest and closest place on the same floor.
    - Total evacuation requires the movement of patients to another healthcare facility.
    - Vertical evacuation requires the movement of patients to the safest lower-level area where movement through horizontal evacuation is not possible.

POP QUIZ 8.8

The OR department manager is notified that there is an electrical fire in the building adjacent to the OR and a code red is in effect. The facilities director tells the OR manager that all procedures are to be halted where feasible and evacuation orders are received. The patients must be evacuated to the first floor of the hospital. The OR is on the third floor. The cases running are as follows:

- A cystoscopy in mid-procedure
- A laparoscopic cholecystectomy case wrapping up
- A total hip arthroplasty that just started
- A tracheostomy for an ICU patient that just started
- Four patients in the holding area
- One patient on the way to the OR suite to undergo a total knee arthroplasty

What type of evacuation would be used in this scenario, and who might the nurse prepare to move first?

PERIOPERATIVE CARDIAC ARREST

During the intraoperative and postoperative period, the patient undergoes substantial physiologic stress. The once-stable patient may decompensate intraoperatively or during the postoperative period, which could lead to complications such as nonfatal myocardial infarction, pulmonary edema, ventricular tachycardia, or patient death.

Assess

Assess the patient for risks associated with cardiac arrest:
- Age (men older than 45 years and women older than 55 years)
- History of myocardial infarction, stroke, CAD, cardiomyopathy, or heart disease
- Obesity or sedentary lifestyle
- Social habits (e.g., smoking, alcohol abuse, illicit drug use)

Confirm

Confirm the presence of the emergency code cart during a cardiac arrest situation.

Evaluate and Ensure

- Evaluate the situation and call for the emergency code cart.
- Ensure the following assistive actions are provided to the anesthesia team and surgeon during a perioperative cardiac arrest:
  - Document all aspects of the process associated with cardiac life support.
  - Facilitate the protection of the sterile table by limiting traffic and movement.
  - Provide assistance with cardiopulmonary resuscitation as directed by the anesthesiologist and/or surgeon.

 NURSING PEARL

The steps of the cardiac event process include the following:
- Retrieve the emergency code cart
- Assist with repositioning the patient
- Perform chest compressions as needed
- Notify the OR manager
- Inform the code leader of tasks performed
- Maintain sterility of the field and surgical counts
- Control the traffic in the room
- Document all interventions

POP QUIZ 8.9

An 80-year-old woman presents to the OR for a cervical discectomy and is placed in the prone position. The patient has hypertension and a history of myocardial infarction that occurred 5 years ago. The patient is anesthetized, positioned, prepped, and draped. Twenty minutes after the surgical incision is made, the patient develops ventricular tachycardia followed by ventricular fibrillation and cardiac arrest. What should the circulating nurse do first to assist the team in managing the issue?

TRAUMA

- Trauma is associated with blunt force and penetrating injuries. Traumatic injuries affect internal organs, bones, the brain, and other soft tissue. These types of injuries are treated as medical emergencies that may cause direct admission into the OR from the emergency department. They may be caused by catastrophic falls, crushing injuries, motor vehicle accidents, stabbings, and gunshot wounds.
- All perioperative nursing care of the trauma patient is contoured to meet needs associated with the nature of the injury. Equipment, instruments, other medical supplies, and positioning requirements are based on surgeon preference and the needs for the particular case.

Assess

- Assess the patient's history, physical and laboratory data and related documentation, and physical presentation.
- Assess the family's presence and coping mechanisms related to the patient's condition.

- Assess for signs of bleeding.
- Assess according to the following nursing diagnoses related to trauma:
  - Acute pain
  - Anxiety and fear
  - Deficient fluid volume
  - Risk for aspiration
  - Risk for hypothermia
- Obtain as much information as possible if the patient is awake, alert, and oriented.
- Assess the patient using the **ABCDE** primary survey method (Rothrock, 2019):
  - **A**irway assessment
  - **B**reathing and ventilation status
  - **C**irculation assessment and hemorrhage status
  - **D**isability related to neurologic issues
  - **E**xposure to injury requiring a full head-to-toe assessment
- Assess the patient related to the type of trauma:
  - Blunt trauma results from automobile accidents or assaults and may be caused by the following:
    - Airbag being deployed
    - Contact with the steering wheel
    - Direction of the impact and distance associated with ejection from a vehicle
    - Seat belt restraint
  - Penetrating trauma results from gunshot wounds or stabbing and is characterized by the following:
    - Distance from the firearm and the point of contact
    - Length of the blade
    - Number of wounds
    - Type of the firearm, blade, or sharp object used

Confirm

- Confirm the method of patient transfer due to positioning to minimize patient injury related to the type of procedure.
- Confirm that all equipment specific to the procedure is available and in the perioperative suite.

Evaluate and Ensure

- Evaluate the need for blood transfusion products, radiology personnel, blood salvage technical support, special instrumentation and equipment, and specialty OR table.
- Evaluate the need for warmed fluids, irrigants, and forced-air warming to promote normothermia.
- Ensure all necessary equipment is available and that personnel associated with the procedure are in the surgical suite and ready to receive the patient.
- Ensure that the following is operational:
  - Equipment for the procedure
  - OR table and positioning equipment
  - Oxygen supply and tanks
  - Suction
- Ensure that the trauma team time-out is performed and includes the following:
  - Arrival situation report on the patient(s) and briefing to the team by the leader
  - Prioritization of the patient needs based upon the assessment
  - Report of the number of inbound patients
  - Summary of the treatment
  - Team debrief

 POP QUIZ 8.10

An 80-year-old female presents to the OR for a cervical fusion following a motor vehicle crash involving three cars. The patient is hypertensive and has a history of myocardial infarction that occurred 7 years prior. The patient is anesthetized, positioned, prepped, and draped. What type of trauma is this, and what should the circulating nurse do next?

RESOURCES

American Association of Nurse Anesthesiology. (2018). *Latex allergy management.* https://www.aana.com/docs/default-source/practice-aana-com-web-documents-(all)/professional-practice-manual/latex-allergy-management.pdf?sfvrsn=9c0049b1_8

American Society of Anesthesiologists. (2013). Practice guidelines for management of the difficult airway: An updated report by the American Society of Anesthesiologists Task Force on management of the difficult airway. *Anesthesiology, 118*(2), 251–270. https://pubs.asahq.org/anesthesiology/article/118/2/251/13535/Practice-Guidelines-for-Management-of-the

American Society of Regional Anesthesia and Pain Medicine. (2020). *Checklist for treatment of local anesthetic systemic toxicity.* https://www.asra.com/guidelines-articles/guidelines/guideline-item/guidelines/2020/11/01/checklist-for-treatment-of-local-anesthetic-systemic-toxicity

Association for periOperative Registered Nurses. (2021a). *EP4 verifying medication labels (NPSG.01.01.01).* https://www.aornguidelines.org/joint-commission/program/46082/standard/46089/ep/543411

Association for periOperative Registered Nurses. (2021b). *Environment of care. Recommendation 3, Guidelines for perioperative practice.* Author.

Association for periOperative Registered Nurses. (2021c). *Environment of care. Recommendation 4, Guidelines for perioperative practice.* Author.

Association for periOperative Registered Nurses. (2021d). *Environment of care. Recommendation 5, Guidelines for perioperative practice.* Author.

Association for periOperative Registered Nurses. (2021e). *Environment of care. Recommendation 7, Guidelines for perioperative practice.* Author.

Association for periOperative Registered Nurses. (2021f). *Environment of care. Recommendation 8, Guidelines for perioperative practice.* Author.

Association for periOperative Registered Nurses. (2021g). *Environment of care. Recommendation 10, Guidelines for perioperative practice.* Author.

Association for periOperative Registered Nurses. (2021h). *Environment of care. Recommendation 11, Guidelines for perioperative practice.* Author.

Association for periOperative Registered Nurses. (2021i). *Laser safety: Recommendation 1—precautions to mitigate hazards, Guidelines for perioperative practice.* Author.

Association for periOperative Registered Nurses. (2021j). *Local anesthesia. Recommendation 3, Guidelines for perioperative practice.* Author.

Association for periOperative Registered Nurses. (2021k). *Patient skin antisepsis, Guidelines for perioperative practice.* Author.

Association of Surgical Technologists. (2018). *Guidelines for best practices for treatment of anaphylactic reaction in the surgical patient.* https://www.ast.org/uploadedFiles/Main_Site/Content/About_Us/Guideline_Anaphylactic_Reaction.pdf

Berkeley, A. V., Ahmed, M. F., & Reardon, J. M. (2021, July 23). *Anaphylaxis in the operating room.* Medscape. https://emedicine.medscape.com/article/2500072-overview

Carlos, G., & Saulan, M. (2018). Robotic emergencies: Are you prepared for a disaster? *AORN Journal, 108*(5), 493–501. https://doi.org/10.1002/aorn.12393

Feldheim, T., Lobo, S., Mallett, J. W., & Le-Wendling, L. (2021). *Local anesthetic systemic toxicity (LAST): A problem-based learning discussion.* https://www.asra.com/guidelines-articles/original-articles/article-item/legacy-b-blog-posts/2021/02/01/local-anesthetic-systemic-toxicity-(last)-a-problem-based-learning-discussion

Fitzgerald, M., Reilly, S., Smit, D. V., Kim, Y., Mathew, J., Boo, E., Alqahtani, A., Chowdhury, S., Darez, A., Mascarenhas, J. B., O'Keeffe, F., Noonan, M., Nickson, C., Marquez, M., Li, W. A., Zhang, Y. L., Williams, K., . . . Mitra, B. (2019). The world health organization trauma checklist versus trauma team time-out: A perspective. *Emergency Medicine Australasia, 31*(5), 882–885. https://doi.org/10.1111/1742-6723.13306

Franklin, B. (1735, February 4). *Protection of towns from fire.* The Pennsylvania Gazette.

Garvey, L. H., Dewachter, P., Hepner, D. L., Mertes, P. M., Voltolini, S., Clarke, R., Cooke, P., Garcez, T., Guttormsen, A. B., Ebo, D. G., Hopkins, P. M., Khan, D. A., Kopac, P., Krøigaard, M., Laguna, J. J., Marshall, S., Platt, P., Rose, M., Sabato, V., . . . Kolawole, H. (2019). Management of suspected immediate perioperative allergic reactions: An international overview and consensus recommendations. *British Journal of Anaesthesia Management, 123*(1), E50–E64. https://doi.org/10.1016/j.bja.2019.04.044

Kollmeier, B. R., Boyette, L. C., Beecham, G. B., Desai, N. M., Khetarpal, S. (2021, August 15). *Difficult airway.* StatPearls. https://www.ncbi.nlm.nih.gov/books/NBK470224/

Malignant Hyperthermia Association of the United States. (2021). *MHAUS recommendations.* https://www.mhaus.org/healthcare-professionals/mhaus-recommendations/

Neal, J. M., Neal, E. J., & Weinberg, G. L. (2021). American society of regional anesthesia and pain medicine local anesthetic systemic toxicity checklist: 2020 version. *Regional Anesthesia & Pain Medicine, 46*(1), 81–82. https://doi.org/10.1136/rapm-2020-101986

Occupational Safety and Health Administration. (n.d.). *Surgical suite: Common safety and health topics*. U.D. Department of Labor, Occupational Safety and Health Administration. https://www.osha.gov/SLTC/etools/hospital/surgical/surgical.html

Rothrock, J. C. (2019). *Alexander's care of the patient in surgery* (16th ed.). Elsevier Health Sciences Division.

PROFESSIONAL ACCOUNTABILITY

OVERVIEW

- Society deems nurses accountable both individually and collectively for delivering quality care.
- The nurse, as a professional, is expected to provide exemplary care beyond the "it's just a job" mentality.
- Nursing as a profession requires the nurse's continuous engagement in professional development to demonstrate a personal commitment to delivering quality care above the expected standard.

ETHICAL AND PROFESSIONAL STANDARDS

Perioperative nurses adhere to the ethical guidelines and professional standards put forth by the ANA and the AORN.

 ALERT!

The premise of safety culture is that systems, not individuals, are to blame for healthcare errors. Promoting a culture of safety balances delivering quality care at the required standard with holding individuals accountable when there is a conscious deviation from the standard.

ANA Code of Ethics

According to the ANA *Code of Ethics for Nurses*, *accountability* is the professional responsibility that an individual nurse has for the patient, public, and health-care organization to follow the scope and standards of nursing practice.

AORN Standards of Perioperative Nursing and the ANA Code of Ethics Alignment

- AORN's perioperative explications align with the ANA Code of Ethics.
- Descriptions of the perioperative nurse's role in relation to each Code of Ethics Interpretive Statement are as follows:
  - 1.1 Respect for Human Dignity
    - Respect the patient's decision for surgery and wishes related to advance directives and end-of-life decisions.
    - Use restraint only when the patient is in a position to harm the self or others.
  - 1.2 Relationship to Patients
    - Provide care to each patient that is consistent and free of prejudicial behavior.
  - 1.3 Nature of Health Problems
    - Provide nursing care that is comprehensive and meets the needs of all patients in a dignified manner.
  - 1.4 Right to Self-Determination
    - Observe the patient's right to autonomy, dignity, and human rights in the perioperative setting through the effective use of informed consent and patient education about the procedure.
  - 1.5 Relationships with Colleagues and Others
    - Ensure that interactions with colleagues/other professionals are done with professionalism and respect for their differences.
  - 2.1 Primacy of Patient Interest
    - Engage in patient advocacy and autonomy related to care decisions.

(continued)

AORN Standards of Perioperative Nursing and the ANA Code of Ethics Alignment *(continued)*

- 2.2 Conflict of Interest for Nurses
  - ○ Do not solicit gifts, gratuities, or any other items of value for services performed.
- 2.3 Collaboration
  - ○ Collaborate with the surgical team to promote positive patient outcomes and to enhance effective communication.
- 2.4 Professional Boundaries
  - ○ Work to avoid unprofessional behavior and recognize personal nurse–patient boundaries.
- 3.1 Privacy
  - ○ Ensure that the patient's body is not needlessly exposed, traffic is minimized, and the doors to the surgical suite are closed.
- 3.2 Confidentiality
  - ○ Protect the patient's medical record by closing the content on the screen or covering the patient's chart.
- 3.3 Protection of Participants in Research
  - ○ Ensure that qualified people are performing research, the patient's rights are safeguarded, and appropriate documentation is present on the chart (i.e., informed consent).
- 3.4 Standards and Review Mechanisms
  - ○ Adhere to AORN's Standards of Professional Performance.
  - ○ Promote a culture of safety.
- 3.5 Acting on Questionable Practice
  - ○ Use the reporting mechanisms within the organization to report questionable practices and unsafe situations.
- 3.6 Addressing Impaired Practice
  - ○ Act as the patient advocate and report instances where impairment of the practitioner may compromise patient safety.
- 4.1 Acceptance of Accountability and Responsibility
  - ○ Delegate tasks and duties to appropriately trained staff within the surgical suite and perioperative unit.
- 4.2 Accountability for Nursing Judgment and Action
  - ○ Practice within the scope and standards issued by ANA and AORN.
- 4.3 Responsibility for Nursing Judgment and Action
  - ○ Assume responsibility for completing continuing education, competency assessment, and additional professional learning.
- 4.4 Delegation of Nursing Activities
  - ○ Act only within the assigned role and delegate tasks only to those who have been appropriately trained for the task.
- 5.1 Moral Self-Respect
  - ○ Work to promote a positive image of nursing and an environment free of abuse.
  - ○ Foster empowerment and team cohesiveness.
- 5.2 Professional Growth and Maintenance of Competency
  - ○ Avoid taking personal and professional risks.
  - ○ Model positive health behaviors.
  - ○ Seek education about current practices and healthcare trends.
- 5.3 Wholeness of Character
  - ○ Be open and genuine in all interactions, and offer opinions based solely on scientific principles and evidence-based practices.
- 5.4 Preservation of Integrity
  - ○ Participate in risk-management and waste-reduction efforts.
- 6.1 Influence of the Environment on Moral Virtues and Values
  - ○ Maintain an environment of mutual respect with the patient and other team members.
- 6.2 Influence of the Environment on Ethical Obligations
  - ○ Follow the practice guidelines for unsafe practices, adhere to policies and procedures, and promote a positive work environment.

- 6.3 Responsibility for Healthcare Environment
  - Promote a culture that is blame free, free from harassment, and conducive to learning and safety.
- 7.1 Advancing the Profession
  - Contribute to the profession through leadership and presence in professional organizations.
- 8.1 Health as a Universal Right
  - Collaborate with elected officials, public health organizations, and other healthcare-related entities to promote the health and well-being of the community.
- 8.2 Collaboration for Health and Human Rights
  - Address health disparities.
  - Integrate patients' cultural differences in the plan of care.
- 9.1 Assertion of Values
  - Maintain memberships in national organizations.
  - Apply a safety-first approach to caring for the patient.
  - Stay current on evidence-based guidelines and practices through the reading of journals and professional literature.

POP QUIZ 9.1

A 75-year-old patient is transported to the surgical suite for a right hip arthroplasty. During the administration of spinal anesthesia, the nurse takes steps to keep the patient covered. Which of the ANA Code of Ethics actions is the perioperative nurse observing?

NURSING SCOPE OF PRACTICE REQUIREMENTS

- Perioperative nursing scope of practice requirements align with practice requirements issued by the ANA Standards for Excellence, Scope and Standards of Practice, and the AORN-recommended practices.
- Perioperative nursing scope of practice requirements are patient centered and ascribe to a model of care that has four domains.

ANA Standards for Excellence

- The ANA's core message is that nurses should practice to the fullest extent of their licensure and education to improve healthcare access and provide high-quality care to patients.
- The ANA Standards for Excellence is a national initiative used to promote the highest standards and includes the following categories:
  - Finance and operations
  - Leadership
  - Legal compliance and ethics
  - Mission, strategy, and evaluation
  - Public awareness, engagement, and advocacy
  - Resource development

ANA Scope and Standard for Practice

- The ANA Scope and Standard for Practice is a list of standards associated with the competency level of nursing care through the use of critical thinking and the nursing process.
- The standards of professional performance are associated with nursing practice that is
  - Based in evidence
  - Collaborative
  - Culturally sensitive
  - Effectively communicated
  - Environmentally safe
  - Ethical
  - High quality
  - Resource efficient

AORN Guidelines for Perioperative Practice

ALERT!

The perioperative nurse should not delegate beyond the requirements outlined in the state nurse practice act.

- AORN's guidelines are considered the gold standard in evidence-based recommended practices guiding the perioperative nurse in decision-making, providing patient care, and promoting workplace safety.
- The guidelines are updated annually and offer recommendations for practice, development of policies and procedures, and criteria for measuring the competency level of the perioperative nurse.

Four Domains

- The perioperative patient-focused model has four domains:
  - Health system where the care is provided
  - Patient safety
  - Patient's behavior in response to the procedure
  - Patient's physiologic response to operative interventions and invasive procedures

State Licensure and Nurse Practice Acts

- Individual states govern health professional licensure.
- Nurse practice acts are state laws governing nursing practice and providing patient care rules and regulations.
- Nurse practice acts by state can be found on the National Council for the State Boards of Nursing website.
- State legislatures pass nurse practice acts, which define the scope of practice. To protect the public, regulatory bodies then issue rules and regulations based on these laws.
- The Board of Nursing for each state enforces the rules and regulations of nurse practice acts.
- The perioperative nurse must maintain all licensing requirements for the state and adhere to the nurse practice acts associated with each state.

LEGAL AND ETHICAL GUIDELINES FOR PATIENT CARE

- The healthcare industry is highly regulated; therefore, healthcare organizations and individuals must understand and comply with individual state laws and regulations, many of which govern practices related to ethical dilemmas perioperative personnel may face.
- The perioperative nurse works to promote health equity and ensures ethical treatment for all patients.

Health Equity

Care of the patient in the perioperative setting should include the following:
- Consideration of the patient's values, beliefs, and lifestyle choice
- Justice and equal treatment regardless of socioeconomic status, race, education, culture, religion, or age
- Protection of patient's free will and right to choose
- Treatment without prejudice or bias

Perioperative Ethical Dilemmas and Legal Issues

- Perioperative ethical dilemmas are commonly associated with the following:
  - Conflict of interest between the nurse's beliefs and the surgery to be performed
  - Conflicting expectations associated with the patient's needs and surgeon's preferences
  - Pressure to turn over a room faster
  - Witnessing of the signature on informed consent

- There are four major categories of legal issue that may arise concerning perioperative nursing practice:
  - Organ donation and transplantation
  - Quality of life
    - ○ Euthanasia and the right to die
  - Reproductive
    - ○ Abortion and sterilization
  - Research
    - ○ Human experimentation and use of stem cells

Factors Contributing to Legal Issues

Factors contributing to legal issues in the perioperative setting include, but are not limited to, the following:
- Causing a direct patient injury related to deviation from duty or standard of care
- Delivery of a low standard of care
- Deviation from a standard of care or omission of important nursing interventions

Legal and Ethical Benefits Associated With Effective Documentation

- The perioperative nurse has a duty to
  - Accurately document all aspects of patient care during the three phases of the perioperative process.
  - Ensure that all patient medical information is protected.
  - Safeguard the electronic health record or other charting modality by exiting the record and safely filing its contents.
- The permanent legal record should be created using a standardized format and incorporate the use of the standardized terminology provided by the PNDS.

PROMOTING A CULTURE OF SAFETY

- All members of the perioperative team must work to promote a culture of safety.
- National guidelines and recommendations help organizations achieve this goal.
- The ANA Code of Ethics, AORN Guidelines, TJC standards, and engagement on committees and professional organizations contribute to the professional development of the nurse and assist in promoting a culture of safety.

The Nurse's Role in Promoting a Culture of Safety

- AORN's (2015) *Position Statement on a Healthy Perioperative Practice Environment* requires an organization to promote the following:
  - Accountability among all team members
  - Collaborative practice
  - Communication that is respectful, helpful, and useful
  - Encouragement of professional practice
  - Recognition of the contributions made by nursing
  - Shared decision-making
  - The visibility of expert leadership
- The perioperative nurse can promote a culture of safety by doing the following:
  - Accurately interpreting the patient's identity and the procedure to be performed
  - Ensuring all surgical counts are performed according to facility policy to reduce the risk of retained foreign bodies
  - Handling all surgical instrumentation and equipment in a safe manner to prevent injury to the patient or the surgical team members
  - Handling patient's personal property with care and ensuring that all personal effects are safely secured per facility policy

(continued)

The Nurse's Role in Promoting a Culture of Safety *(continued)*

- Promoting a culture of respect, collaboration, and teamwork
- Protecting the patient from accidental fall or injury during transport to the surgical suite and transfer to the surgical table by ensuring adequate personnel is available to assist
- Reporting all adverse events and changes to the patient's condition
- Safely securing and preparing all specimens per facility policy

 NURSING PEARL

Use this mnemonic **CCARES** to remember how to promote a culture of safety:

- **C**ollaborate with the team
- **C**ommunicate effectively
- **A**ccept responsibility for your actions
- **R**ecognize the contributions of others
- **E**ncourage one another
- **S**hare in the decision-making

ANA Code of Ethics

- The ANA *Code of Ethics for Nurses with Interpretative Statements* calls upon employers in both academic and clinical settings to foster a workplace free of incivility, lateral and workplace violence, and bullying.
- The perioperative nurse has a responsibility to the self and others to use best practices related to the management and report of issues associated with incivility, lateral or workplace violence, and bullying, including the following:
  - Collaborate with all team members through open dialogue and sharing of information in a timely manner.
  - Encourage a nonpunitive work environment.
  - Maintain a detailed written account of incidents.
  - Participate in workplace violence prevention education programs and postevent debriefings.
  - Provide assistance when needed.
  - Recognize one's own actions in a situation.
  - Rely on facts and refrain from spreading gossip or rumors.
  - Remain open to the ideas of others.
  - Respond to incivility in a respectful manner and report using the appropriate channels.
  - Support team members who have been a target of uncivil behaviors or workplace violence.
  - Treat all team members with respect and dignity.
  - Use clear and civil communication across all mediums (written, verbal, social media, etc.).
  - Work to incorporate personal wellness strategies to decrease stress.

AORN Recommendations

- AORN recommends that organizational leadership implement best practices to promote a safety culture. Best practices should promote respect, honesty, collaboration, and accountability among individuals and teams across healthcare disciplines. They should also facilitate effective communication and empower perioperative personnel to speak up. Examples include the following:
  - Interdisciplinary team members participate in a standardized approach to handoff communication, including verification using readback methods.
  - Perioperative personnel comply with the protocol for patient preprocedure checks and time-out processes. Each team member participates and contributes.
- AORN encourages employers to offer structured orientation as a means to encourage a safety culture.
  - Perioperative residency programs assist in decreasing the theory-to-practice gap and should include preceptor education, training, and evaluation.
  - Precepted competency-based orientation programs should be measurable and provided to perioperative RNs and surgical technologists upon hire.

TJC Standards

- TJC highlights key standards integral to an organization's commitment to safety culture.

- TJC issues NPSGs annually to highlight healthcare-related adverse events and practice issues in the following practice areas:
  - Ambulatory healthcare
  - Behavioral healthcare
  - Critical access hospital
  - Home care
  - Hospital
  - Laboratory
  - Nursing care center
  - Office-based surgery center
- The following are NPSGs associated with the perioperative setting:
  - Identifying patient safety risks
  - Identifying patients correctly
  - Improving staff communication
  - Preventing infection
  - Preventing mistakes in surgery
  - Safety associated with medication administration
  - Utilization of alarms
- These standards from TJC require that the organizational leadership implement the following practices:
  - Nonpunitive internal mechanisms for reporting near or actual adverse events to encourage reporting and increase opportunities for shared learning
  - Policies that prohibit intimidating behaviors
  - Procedures for promoting a safety culture and performing assessments through the use of validated surveys to identify areas for improvement
  - Risk assessment approaches emphasizing that systems, not individuals, are the blame for near or actual events

 POP QUIZ 9.2

A circulating nurse contributes to a medication error. The circulating nurse reports the mistake through the safety event system. An RCA ensues. The collaborative RCA findings point to an inadequate electronic medical record fail-safe mechanism for alerting healthcare professionals to overdose or underdose medication. The processes described in this scenario illustrate which key concepts around safety culture?

PROFESSIONAL GROWTH AND ACCOUNTABILITY

- Ongoing engagement in professional growth and accountability is a foundational aspect of nursing practice.
- Maintaining personal accountability to the self and others, participating in membership in national organizations, obtaining specialty certification, and engaging in professional development activities are ways that the perioperative nurse can grow professionally.

Accountability

AORN highlights the professional practice of the perioperative RN within the context of accountability to illustrate the importance of a nurse's behavior. The RN is accountable to the patient, team, and organization for performing at a level that is considered standard of care.

- Perioperative leadership teams have moral and legal responsibilities to identify risks and implement actions to prevent harm.
- Perioperative nursing is a specialty that requires ongoing professional development to continually increase knowledge and skills.
- Perioperative personnel who lack accountability for behavior may cause patient harm and patient dissatisfaction with the quality of care.

Membership in National Organizations

AORN encourages membership in professional organizations. These associations provide evidence-based guidelines and standards for patient safety and clinical issues. Examples of professional organizations in which nurses may seek membership include the following:

- ANA
  - https://www.nursingworld.org/membership/joinANA/
- ASPAN
  - https://www.aspan.org/
- APND
  - https://www.anpd.org/
- APIC
  - https://apic.org/
- AORN
  - https://www.aorn.org/
- NLN
  - http://www.nln.org/
- IAHCSMM
  - https://www.iahcsmm.org/

Professional Development

- AORN strongly encourages professional development and specifically endorses the value of specialty certification.
- Perioperative nursing specialty certification demonstrates to the public, patients, colleagues, and employers that nurses are committed to delivering the highest quality care possible.
  - Perioperative nursing specialty certification:
    - Is a formal means to recognize nurses' knowledge, skills, and experience.
    - Measures the nurse's knowledge objectively, validating at a standard level the knowledge necessary to provide high-quality care.
  - Perioperative leadership teams should:
    - Display the credentials of certified perioperative RNs.
    - Market the RNs' professional certification to the public to demonstrate alignment with AORN's message of seeking licensure, accreditation, certification, and education to promote patient safety and provide protection to the public.
    - Support RNs in obtaining certification.
- The perioperative nurse should utilize the resources available at the place of work, in the community, and through professional organizations to enhance professional growth.

QUALITY IMPROVEMENT USING EVIDENCE-BASED PRACTICE

The perioperative nurse should remain engaged in quality improvement initiatives and incorporate the use of evidence-based practice guidelines and recommendations in all facets of practice.

Engagement in Evidence-Based Practice

Evidence-based practices are the foundation of the AORN guidelines. Perioperative personnel should use the guidelines to inform quality patient care and quality improvement strategies, including the implementation of policies based on best practices. Examples include standardization in the following areas:

- Counting process
- Hand-off approach
- Patient identification
- Patient normothermia protocols
- Time-out processes

Quality Improvement Agencies

Quality improvement agencies decrease healthcare costs, enhance provider experience, and improve population health, patient experiences, or patient outcomes. Quality improvement agencies include the following:

- Agency for Healthcare Research and Quality
- Institute for Healthcare Improvement
- TJC Center for Transforming Healthcare

Methods for Quality Improvement Engagement

- Common process or quality improvement models used in the perioperative setting include, but are not limited to, the following:
  - **PICO** framework for developing clinical questions:
    - Patient/problem (What is the issue?)
    - Intervention (What is the intervention?)
    - Comparison (What are the alternatives?)
    - Outcome (What is the desired outcome?)
  - Plan-Do-Study-Act
    - The *PDSA* is a four-step problem-solving cycle that is used to implement a plan for change.
    - The PDSA cycle enables organizations to test changes on a small scale, build on what was learned, and maximize processes for larger-scale implementation.
  - RCA
    - The *RCA* is a critique of processes following an adverse event used to mitigate future risk.
  - Six Sigma
    - *Six Sigma* is a systematic process for improving workplace efficiency.
- Participation in quality-of-care activities helps the perioperative nurse to stay engaged and promote lasting change by
  - Advocating for changes to processes that impede a safe and effective workflow.
  - Attending meetings and serving on committees related to quality improvement initiatives.
  - Collecting data on quality improvement initiatives.
  - Identifying and accepting responsibility for ongoing monitoring and evaluation activities within the department.
  - Maintaining knowledge on current practice changes, professional nursing scope of practice responsibilities, delegation restraints, and regulatory standards.
  - Performing quality assessments and RCAs on a routine basis.
- Shared governance fosters quality improvement engagement for the perioperative nurse by
  - Empowering nurses to continuously improve patient care and the work environment.
  - Enhancing collaboration with interprofessional team members to improve patient care.
  - Providing nurses with responsibility, authority, and accountability related to decision-making processes.

RESOURCES

Agency for Healthcare Research and Quality. (n.d.). *Patient safety and quality improvement.* https://www.ahrq.gov/patient-safety/index.html

American Nurses Association. (2015a). *American nurses association position statement on incivility, bullying, and workplace violence.* https://www.nursingworld.org/~49d6e3/globalassets/practiceandpolicy/nursing-excellence/incivility-bullying-and-workplace-violence--ana-position-statement.pdf

American Nurses Association. (2015b). *Code of ethics for nurses with interpretive statements.* https://www.nursingworld.org/practice-policy/nursing-excellence/ethics/code-of-ethics-for-nurses/coe-view-only/

American Nurses Association. (n.d.). *Scope of practice.* https://www.nursingworld.org/practice-policy/scope-of-practice/

Association for periOperative Registered Nurses. (2015a). *Exhibit A: Historical perspectives on the AORN standards, competency statements, and certification. AORN standards.* https://www.aorn.org/guidelines/clinical-resources/aorn-standards

Association for periOperative Registered Nurses. (2015b). Healthy perioperative practice environment. Position statements. https://www.aorn.org/guidelines/clinical-resources/position-statements

Association for periOperative Registered Nurses. (2015c). *Position statement on a healthy perioperative practice environment. Position statements.* https://www.aorn.org/guidelines/clinical-resources/position-statements

Association for periOperative Registered Nurses. (2016). *Perioperative nursing certification. Position statements.* https://www.aorn.org/guidelines/clinical-resources/position-statements

Association for periOperative Registered Nurses. (2017). *AORN's perioperative explications for the ANA code of ethics for nurses with interpretative statements.* https://www.aorn.org/guidelines/clinical-resources/code-of-ethics

Association for periOperative Registered Nurses. (2018). *Position statement on orientation of the registered nurse and surgical technologist to the perioperative setting. Position statements.* https://www.aorn.org/guidelines/clinical-resources/position-statements

Association for periOperative Registered Nurses. (2019). *AORN position statement on perioperative registered nurse residency programs. Position statements.* https://www.aorn.org/guidelines/clinical-resources/position-statements

Association for periOperative Registered Nurses. (2021a). *About: Guidelines for perioperative practice.* https://www.aorn.org/guidelines/about-aorn-guidelines

Association for periOperative Registered Nurses. (2021b). *Guideline for a safe environment of care, Guidelines for perioperative practice.* Author.

Clement, N. (2013). *Ethical and legal issues in perioperative nursing. Nursing ethics.* Pearson India. https://learning.oreilly.com/library/view/nursing-ethics/9788131773345/xhtml/chapter030.xhtml

Institute for Healthcare Improvement. (n.d.). *Quality improvement essentials toolkit.* [Toolkit]. http://www.ihi.org/resources/Pages/Tools/Quality-Improvement-Essentials-Toolkit.aspx

The Joint Commission. (2018). *Patient safety systems. Comprehensive accreditation manual.* Joint Commission Resources.

Joint Commission Center for Transforming Healthcare. (n.d.). *Who we are.* https://www.centerfortransforminghealthcare.org/who-we-are/

Kutney-Lee, A., Germack, H., Hatfield, L., Kelly, S., Maguire, P., Dierkes, A., Guidice, M. D., & Aiken, L. H. (2016). Nurse engagement in shared governance and patient and nurse outcomes. *The Journal of Nursing Administration, 46*(11), 605–612. https://doi.org/10.1097/NNA.0000000000000412

Rothrock, J. C. (2019). *Alexander's care of the patient in surgery* (16th ed.). Elsevier Health Sciences Division.

10

ANSWERS TO POP QUIZZES AND UNFOLDING SCENARIOS

CHAPTER 2

UNFOLDING SCENARIO 2.1A

Assessment of the documentation associated with the surgery is required (e.g., history and physical, laboratory and diagnostic results, informed consent, and anesthesia consent).

POP QUIZ 2.1

The anesthesiologist should be made aware that the surgical site is not marked, and the nerve block will need to be delayed. The surgeon will need to be contacted and asked to mark the patient.

UNFOLDING SCENARIO 2.1B

Alert the team that the time-out has not been performed. Ask all members of the team to pause so that this important action can be completed.

UNFOLDING SCENARIO 2.1C

Alert the team that the patient has not been securely strapped. Ask the scrub technician to carefully move away. Place the strap across the thighs. The belt must be out of the way of the surgical field.

POP QUIZ 2.2

The circulating nurse should alert the anesthesiologist and the surgeon right away. The surgical site marking should be consistent with the patient's confirmation of the procedure and the contents of the surgical consent.

POP QUIZ 2.3

The circulating nurse should identify the procedure performed, the drains (if used), and the need for blood products and blood salvage.

UNFOLDING SCENARIO 2.1D

Alert the anesthesiologist and page the surgeon back to the OR suite. The patient is showing signs of hypervolemia.

UNFOLDING SCENARIO 2.2A

Assess patient's range of motion related to positioning in lithotomy. Confer with the surgeon and the anesthesiologist on the patient's refusal of blood products. Consider the use of cell salvage.

UNFOLDING SCENARIO 2.2B

- Off the field
  - Call for the emergency cart and blood salvage device.
  - Call for massive transfusion equipment and products if there is a trauma or massive hemorrhage.
  - Check the suction and be sure that it is operational and that there are multiple empty canisters ready.
  - Ensure that there is warm sterile saline to dispense to the surgical field.
- On the field
  - Anticipate the surgeon's needs.
  - Monitor the use of sponges or towels and be sure that what was placed in the cavity is removed.
  - Note the canister volume during the transition. If normal saline irrigation is used, take the added volume into account in the suction canister volume when anesthesia wants to know how much blood has been lost.
  - Prepare the room to convert to a fully open procedure.
  - Rapidly provide instrumentation, sutures, and stapling devices as requested by the surgeon.

UNFOLDING SCENARIO 2.2C

- Assist anesthesia personnel in the appropriate laboratory specimen acquisition (i.e., type, screen, and cross) and call the lab personnel to advise that a stat result is needed.
- Follow facility policy and procedure associated with critical lab procurement and transport of the blood specimens to the laboratory.
- Provide assistive service to the surgeon and other personnel at the sterile field.

CHAPTER 3

UNFOLDING SCENARIO 3A

Assessment of the documentation associated with the surgery is required, including history and physical, laboratory and diagnostic results, surgical consent, and anesthesia consent.

UNFOLDING SCENARIO 3B

The following nursing diagnoses would be considered for this patient:
- Acute pain
- Impaired physical mobility
- Risk for ineffective tissue perfusion
- Risk for infection

UNFOLDING SCENARIO 3C

The nurse should plan for and anticipate the need for a large specimen box and confer with the physician on the disposition of the limb. *Note:* Some patients may request to retrieve the limb due to cultural practices.

POP QUIZ 3.1

Outcome statement: The patient is free from signs and symptoms of electrical injury.

POP QUIZ 3.2

PNDS is integrated through perioperative documentation to:

1. Detect the risks associated with patient care.
2. Identify deficiencies in documentation.
3. Improve how electronic documentation is done through the use of preset fields.
4. Standardize documentation through the use of a universal language.

UNFOLDING SCENARIO 3D

The next action is to complete the surgical count of sponges and sharps used in the procedure.

UNFOLDING SCENARIO 3E

Ensure that the patient's leg is fully cleaned, and a new gown placed on the patient prior to moving the patient to the bed.

CHAPTER 4

UNFOLDING SCENARIO 4A

The perioperative nurse should ask for the team to pause and perform the time-out process.

UNFOLDING SCENARIO 4B

The perioperative nurse should post the x-rays and MRI images for display. All images and diagnostic results needed for the surgery should be posted where all team members can see without obstruction.

POP QUIZ 4.1

Padding should be placed to support the occiput, scapulae, arms, elbows, thoracic vertebrae, sacrum/coccyx, and heels.

UNFOLDING SCENARIO 4C

- Elbows/arms
- Occiput: with a foam or gel headrest
- Operative leg: if in a holder, then it needs to be padded and secured. Check circulation prior to draping.
- Non-operative leg: securely position as directed by the surgeon and pad the heel.

UNFOLDING SCENARIO 4D

- Ensure that all fluids have been dried from the floor to prevent slip and fall.
- Ensure that the foot of the bed has been elevated and made ready to move the patient's legs back to anatomical position.
- Remain at the side of the bed to assist anesthesia personnel during the patient's emergence from anesthesia.
- Return the safety strap to the patient, if it has been moved during the procedure or following surgical intervention.

POP QUIZ 4.2

The scrub nurse and the circulating nurse should begin a full search of the surgical field and around the field, respectively. While the surgeon continues to work, all of the unnecessary sharps and sponges should be removed from the field. The contents of the kick bucket, the floor, the bottoms of staff shoes, under the furniture, and the room trash (with a magnet if needed) should be evaluated by the circulator. Once those steps are complete, and it is found that the needle is still missing, the surgeon should be notified as radiology may need to be called to assess whether or not the sharp is retained within the body cavity.

POP QUIZ 4.3

The circulating nurse should alert the scrub person that the gown is compromised, and the scrub person should be advised to remove the gown, re-scrub, re-gown, and re-glove.

POP QUIZ 4.4

- Communicate to the team that there is a fire.
- Extinguish the fire, remove the drape, and assess whether there is any additional potential harm to the patient. Once the fire is extinguished, the circulating nurse should replace the damaged drape with a new, sterile one.
- Move the foot pedals to a position that can be seen by the surgeon.

POP QUIZ 4.5

Confirm with the surgeon how the specimen should be sent to pathology and the description of the suture-marked areas.

CHAPTER 5

POP QUIZ 5.1

The nurse should alert the surgeon that assistive personnel cannot be delegated this duty because formal training is required.

UNFOLDING SCENARIO 5A

The circulating nurse should pause and let the visitor know that no one is to move during the time-out. The resident should be asked to move back to the original position.

UNFOLDING SCENARIO 5B

The circulating nurse should immediately go to the resident and assist them into a chair. The nurse should then call the charge nurse to ask for someone to escort the resident out of the OR.

POP QUIZ 5.2

The circulating nurse should ask the HCIR why they are in the room prior to the patient being draped for surgery. If the representative is assisting the scrub person with the assembly of instrumentation, the nurse may permit them to stay. The nurse should remind the representative to maintain a safe distance from the surgical field to avoid contamination.

POP QUIZ 5.3

The nurse should refrain from opening the contents and notify the manager. In this scenario, the nurse cannot approve the use of the cement because its use would violate facility policy and procedure.

CHAPTER 6

POP QUIZ 6.1

The scrub and circulating nurses should have examined the package integrity, size of the graft, and expiration date prior to dispensation to the surgical field. Cross-monitoring, situational awareness, and effective communication could have prevented the error.

UNFOLDING SCENARIO 6A

Answer 1: The allergies should have been communicated and verified prior to the application of the skin prep. The anesthesia provider and the circulator should have communicated the need for at least one additional person to facilitate positioning of the patient.

Answer 2: The circulating nurse should have confirmed that the strap was secure on both sides and should have communicated that there was pooling of the skin prep solution.

UNFOLDING SCENARIO 6B

The skin assessment postoperatively should be documented. The nurse should also follow facility policy on the filing of an incident report and any notes associated with adverse events or unplanned activities as per facility policy.

POP QUIZ 6.2

The nurse should communicate the findings to the surgeon, who will determine the course of action related to the surgery and document the findings in the patient's health record. The anesthesia team may need to delay induction until the surgeon assesses the patient's heel and makes a decision on whether or not the surgery can be performed.

CHAPTER 7

UNFOLDING SCENARIO 7A

The neutral zone is used to reduce the incidence of sharps injuries.

To protect the patient from microbial contamination, the scrub personnel should remove the knife from the surgical field and safely hand it off to the circulating nurse because it is now contaminated. Next, the scrub personnel should let the circulator know that there is a need for a drape and alert the surgeon that there is a breach in the existing drape. The scrub personnel should also orient the surgeon to the instrument mat and explain that it will be used as the neutral zone for the remainder of the surgical case.

UNFOLDING SCENARIO 7B

The circulating nurse should advise the surgical scrub person who is using alcohol-based hand antisepsis products that this should be performed with the same rigor as the scrubbing performed by using a scrub brush and sponge, attending to each of the four sides of the hands and fingers on both hands.

The circulating nurse should remind the relief nurse to use facility- and FDA-approved hand lotion in the clinical setting to avoid unintentional microbial spread or allergic reactions from patients.

UNFOLDING SCENARIO 7C

The scrub person should follow the facility policy for blood-borne pathogen exposure after notifying the surgeon of the issue. If the scrub person is actively bleeding, it is necessary to confine and contain the bleed away from the sterile field to avoid microbial exposure to the patient and cross-contamination of the sterile field.

UNFOLDING SCENARIO 7D

Because the surgeon has been notified that there is a sterilization issue, and the only other similar tray is in use, the nurse should review the manufacturer's instructions related to IUSS and then proceed with sterilization according to the manufacturer's parameters for steam sterilization.

UNFOLDING SCENARIO 7E

The documentation for IUSS should be complete and include the date, time, instrument(s), cycle parameters, monitoring results, operator information, patient identification, reason for IUSS, and type of cycle used.

All sharps should be removed from the sterile field after the end of the procedure and final count. All sharps should be removed from instrumentation to protect sterile processing staff from sharps injuries. Sharps should be removed using another instrument and not by hand.

POP QUIZ 7.1

Following the facility policies and procedures related to instrument tracking prevents delays and improves communication on the status of instruments in transit.

POP QUIZ 7.2

Assess all areas of the surgical suite for cleanliness before opening sterile contents for the case.

POP QUIZ 7.3

The term for moisture in a pack or tray is "wet pack." The circulating nurse should remove the tray from use before the scrub person reaches for it. The circulating nurse should notify the sterile processing leadership team or designated personnel so that an investigation ensues to determine the cause or causes of the moisture.

CHAPTER 8

POP QUIZ 8.1

The patient is exhibiting signs of anaphylaxis related to the isosulfan blue dye injection. The circulating nurse should call for help and the emergency code cart and then immediately move to the head of the bed to support the patient and the anesthesia personnel. The surgery will come to a pause, a secure airway will be established and confirmed, and the anesthesiologist will order medication to counteract the reaction.

POP QUIZ 8.2

The primary responsibilities of the perioperative circulating nurse in this scenario are as follows:
- Assist the anesthesia personnel as needed.
- Complete a surgical count when it is feasible to do so.
- Open all additional equipment, instruments, sharps, and sponges as requested by the surgeon.
- Provide warmed sterile saline for irrigation of the abdominal cavity.
- Shut off the light source and insufflation machine.
- Turn on the OR lights and room lights.

POP QUIZ 8.3

The perioperative circulating nurse should remain at the head of the bed to provide support for the patient and the anesthesia team as directed by the anesthesiologist of record.

POP QUIZ 8.4

The nurse should cover all cords with facility-approved cord covers and ensure that pathways are not obstructed around the surgical field and within the suite.

POP QUIZ 8.5

The nurse should call for help and ask that the emergency code cart be brought into the suite. The nurse should then begin to open supplies as ordered. The nurse should also coordinate with anesthesia personnel and be prepared to call the blood bank for blood products.

POP QUIZ 8.6

This patient is likely experiencing LAST. The circulating nurse should alert the surgeon that the patient appears confused and that he is bradycardic, call for help to retrieve the rescue kit and emergency code cart, and monitor the airway.

POP QUIZ 8.7

The nurse should call for additional help and the emergency code cart, then begin dilution of dantrolene sodium. MHAUS recommends a starting dose of dantrolene at 2.5 mg/kg. Reconstitution of dantrolene will depend upon the brand used. If the facility has a separate MH cart, that should be brought into the surgical suite.

POP QUIZ 8.8

Vertical evacuation is necessary as the OR manager has been advised that all patients must be moved to the first floor. The nurse should plan to move the ambulatory patients first. The nurse should always follow the facility fire evacuation plan when moving patients.

POP QUIZ 8.9

The nurse should assist in moving the patient to the supine position to maximize chest compressions and aid with compressions as directed.

POP QUIZ 8.10

The type of trauma is a blunt force. The patient was involved in a motor vehicle accident that resulted in a cervical injury. The circulating nurse should call for a time-out just before the surgeon makes an incision.

CHAPTER 9

POP QUIZ 9.1

3.1 Privacy: Ensure that the patient's body is not needlessly exposed, traffic is minimized, and the doors to the surgical suite are closed.

POP QUIZ 9.2

The organization had mechanisms for reporting the error and completed an RCA. Additionally, the organization's approach was nonpunitive, evaluating system failures rather than blaming the individual. This scenario describes an organization that employed principles of safety culture.

APPENDIX: ABBREVIATIONS

AATB	American Association of Tissue Banks
ACE	assess, confirm, evaluate and ensure
ADPIE	assessment, diagnosis, outcome identification, planning, implementation of interventions, evaluation data
ANA	American Nurses Association
ANPIE	*See* ADPIE
AORN	Association of periOperative Registered Nurses
APIC	Association for Professionals in Infection Control and Epidemiology
APND	Association for Nursing Professional Development
APRN	advanced practice registered nurse
aPTT	activated partial thromboplastin time
ASA	American Society of Anesthesiologists
ASPAN	American Society of PeriAnesthesia Nurses
ATLS	advanced trauma life support
BMP	basic metabolic panel
CAD	coronary artery disease
CBC	complete blood count
CCI	Competency and Credentialing Institute
CDC	Centers for Disease Control
CHG	chlorhexidine gluconate
CJD	Creutzfeldt-Jakob disease
CKD	chronic kidney disease
CMS	Centers for Medicaid and Medical Services
CNOR	Certified Perioperative Nurse
COPD	chronic obstructive pulmonary disease
CRNA	Certified Registered Nurse Anesthetist
CT	computed tomography
DIC	disseminated intravascular coagulation
DM	diabetes mellitus
EKG	electrocardiogram
ESU	electrosurgical unit
FDA	U.S. Food and Drug Administration
HAI	healthcare-associated infection
HCIR	healthcare industry representative
HCT	hematocrit
HGB	hemoglobin
HEPA	high-efficiency particulate air
HIPAA	Health Insurance Portability and Accountability Act
IAHCSMM	International Association of Healthcare Central Service Material Management
ICD	implanted cardioverter defibrillator
IFU	instructions for use
INR	international normalized ratio
IUSS	immediate use of steam sterilization
IV	intravenous

LAST	local anesthetic systemic toxicity
LFT	liver function test
MDRO	multidrug-resistant organisms
MH	malignant hyperthermia
MHAUS	Malignant Hyperthermia Association of the United States
MRSA	methicillin-resistant *Staphylococcus aureus*
MSDS	material safety data sheet
NANDA	North American Nursing Diagnosis Association
NLN	National League for Nursing
NP	nurse practitioner
NPO	nothing by mouth
NPSG	National Patient Safety Goal
OR	operating room
OSA	obstructive sleep apnea
OSHA	Occupational Safety and Health Administration
PA	physician assistant
PACU	postanesthesia care unit
PDSA	Plan-Do-Study-Act
PICO	Patient, Intervention, Comparison, Outcome
PLT	platelets
PNDS	Perioperative Nursing Data Set
PPE	personal protective equipment
PT	prothrombin time
PTT	partial thromboplastin time
RBC	red blood cells
RCA	root cause analysis
RN	registered nurse
RNFA	registered nurse first assistant
SAMPLE	Symptoms, Allergies, Medications, Past medical history, Last oral intake, Events or environment that led to the accident or injury
SBAR	Situation, Background, Assessment, Recommendation
SCIP	Surgical Care Improvement Project
SSI	surgical site infection
TAPE	Type of procedure, Anticipated blood loss, Presence of type and cross match, Evaluation by surgeon
TB	tuberculosis
TJC	The Joint Commission
TSE	transmissible spongiform encephalopathy
WBC	white blood cells

INDEX

Printed in the United States
by Baker & Taylor Publisher Services